THE NOURISHED BRAIN

THE LATEST SCIENCE ON FOOD'S POWER
FOR PROTECTING THE BRAIN FROM ALZHEIMER'S AND DEMENTIA

CHERYL MUSSATTO MS, RD, LD

In loving memory of my parents, Cecil and Shirley.
Your love, support, and dedication to put family first,
shaped our values, beliefs, and who we are today.
Your memory lives on in each of us.

Contents

Foreword   1

Introduction   3

PART 1 BRAIN-HEALTHY SCIENCE

Chapter 1: A Brain Health Crisis   7

Chapter 2: Understanding the Brain   14

Chapter 3: Studies on Food's Role in Brain Health   20

PART 2 BRAIN-HEALTHY NOURISHMENT

Chapter 4: Essential Nutrients for the Brain   28

*Chapter 5: Food for Thought – Brain-Sustaining and
        Brain-Draining Foods*   37

Chapter 6: Meal Planning to Maximize Brain Health   59

Chapter 7: Leading Your Best Brain Healthy Lifestyle   67

PART 3 BRAIN-HEALTHY RECIPES

Chapter 8: Recipes Promoting Brain Health   74

Acknowledgements   108

References   110

Index   116

FOREWORD

I have spent the first 20 years of my career studying the most intricate, complex organ in the body — the brain — and I hope to spend the next 50 doing the same. Its mystery and complexity drew me into the field. Unlocking the brain's secrets is today's greatest scientific challenge. The brain makes us who we are, underlying all our behaviors, feelings, actions, and personality. As a neurologist, I see evidence of this every day; everything the brain does, disease can warp or take away entirely.

Alzheimer's disease is one of those diseases. Its progressive degeneration erases our memories and alters the very person we are as it inevitably progresses to its end stage. The good news is we are living longer healthier lives. Never before have there been more individuals over the age of 65. The bad news is Alzheimer's disease risk is tightly linked to age: 1 in 9 individuals over 65 years and an amazing 1 in 3 over the age 85 have Alzheimer's disease, which affects more than 5 million Americans. This epidemic, which is currently the sixth leading cause of death in the United States, is projected to explode to 14 million by 2050 as the baby boomer generation progresses through retirement.

This is why scientists all over the world are working to find a cure for this disease. Although there are several drugs that can slow cognitive changes, none can stop or reverse the inevitable change that occurs as Alzheimer's progresses. As a neurologist, I focus specifically on finding ways to keep our brains healthy as we age. At first glance, it may seem that this monumental problem is entirely in the hands of scientists.

However, more and more evidence supports lifestyle factors, including diet and exercise, as key contributors to the prevention of

Alzheimer's disease. All the high tech advances, and billions of dollars spent researching this topic, continues to suggest the most reliable and efficacious way to advance your brain health remains in our own hands through the lifestyle choices we make, specifically diet and exercise.

The University of Kansas Alzheimer's Disease Center (KU ADC), one of only 31 nationally designated Alzheimer's Disease Centers in the United States, is working to eliminate the disease through research into curing and preventing Alzheimer's disease. We believe the day will come when we can spot the disease before any memory loss occurs and intervene to stop it entirely. Nevertheless, when that day comes (and certainly until it comes) lifestyle factors will remain an important strategy to maintain your brain health.

It is vital that you understand you have power in this fight to reduce your long-term risk. That is why the KU ADC developed the LEAP! Program (Lifestyle Empowerment for Alzheimer's Prevention) to translate the latest Alzheimer's disease prevention research into actionable recommendations for everyday life. And, it is why Registered Dietitian Cheryl Mussatto has written this book.

Cheryl's easy-to-follow guide for a brain-healthy diet was developed after witnessing the devastation of Alzheimer's disease within her own family. This user-friendly guide provides you with evidence-based nutritional advice to support optimal brain health, including recipes and recommendations for dietary habits to improve your health with a focus on brain health.

This couldn't come at a better time when it is increasingly crucial that we fight back against this increasingly important disease.

Jeffrey M. Burns, M.D., M.S.
Co-Director of the University of Kansas Alzheimer's Disease Center

Edward H. Hashinger, Professor of Medicine
Department of Neurology, University of Kansas Medical Center

INTRODUCTION

My personal experience with Alzheimer's disease began with an unexpected phone call. A woman I've known since childhood called with concerns of my Mom's mental health. Since I, along with my other three siblings, lived at least an hour from our parent's farm, I honestly could not say I had noticed a huge change. Visits back home were regular but not often. Mom was still driving, cooking (at least we thought), paying bills, and taking care of the house. What did she mean, "Had I noticed a change in my mom?"

A quick phone call to my Mom's physician confirmed my fears – Mom had Alzheimer's disease. How did we miss the signs? Or did we? Maybe we each chose to ignore her repetitive questions, heightened anxiety, poor financial decisions, and increased confusion on simple tasks. Maybe we knew something was wrong but wanted to believe that Mom would "get over it." At this time, my Dad was facing his own health problems associated with a condition called normal pressure hydrocephalus he had been diagnosed with years ago and was now showing signs of dementia himself.

Just like millions of other families, we faced this diagnosis with heavy hearts. And so began our long goodbye with our beloved Mom over the next two years before she passed away from complications of Alzheimer's.

The degenerative and irreversible disease of Alzheimer's operates on a level playing field. Alzheimer's seems to strike at random, regardless of socioeconomics, gender, or ethnicity. Worldwide, up to 50 million people are living with some form of dementia, including Alzheimer's and that number is expected to reach a staggering 76 million people around the globe by 2030. On average, people with Alzheimer's live eight to ten years after diagnosis but others may live as long as 20 years. There is no cure at this time.

An Alzheimer's diagnosis means difficult decisions must be made. Each family is different in their approach depending on circumstances. For my siblings and I, these decisions were some of the most challenging and painful we've ever had to make - moving our parents off the farm into senior housing, coordinating in-home caregivers, taking away the car keys, monitoring and managing their medical and financial decisions, occasionally helping them with personal tasks of dressing and toileting, and hardest of all, the emotional toll of having to witness the gradual but steady loss of the Mom and Dad we once knew. It was a life journey none of us wanted to or anticipated to take but was necessary as we honored the parents we deeply loved as best we could.

I asked myself the question of every family that encounters this disease: "Is there something that could have been done to prevent it?"

In this book, I share personal anecdotes from family and friends who have also had to travel this unexpected journey of a loved one diagnosed with Alzheimer's disease. Their stories are part of the millions whose lives have been forever changed by this disease, and I am grateful to have their blessing to share these.

As a Registered Dietitian, I have the privilege of helping people live their healthiest lives through dietary changes. My purpose is to shine a spotlight on the role of food and diet and its possible power to thwart off the clutches of Alzheimer's. Even though the science of using food to stave off Alzheimer's disease is still evolving, it looks promising that long-term changes in how you eat can have a protective effect. Other factors within our control – exercise, keeping socially active, and brain activity will also be addressed.

This book is divided into three parts:

Part 1 will provide an introduction of Alzheimer's disease and dementia with a look at the inner workings of the brain and numerous studies showing a strong correlation between food choices that either nourish or hinder brain health.

Part 2 will guide you through how to create a brain-healthy meal plan by knowing what foods to buy and how often certain foods should be eaten.

Part 3 will provide a compilation of recipes ingredients containing nutrients known to be beneficial for brain health complete with nutritional information. All recipes are simple, delicious and nutritious options for every meal along with snacks that the whole family can enjoy.

PART 1
BRAIN-HEALTY SCIENCE

CHAPTER ONE

A Brain Health Crisis

"The summer of 2010 I'll never forget. Mom was diagnosed with Alzheimer's disease and by January of 2012 she died peacefully surrounded by her family. Between those dates, our family painfully witnessed the disease steal our Mom and we were helpless to stop it. Watching her slip away was the most difficult thing I've had to experience. I could only imagine what she was going through. Mom suffered terribly with extreme anxiety and as I sat with her one day doing my best to comfort and console her, I caught a glimpse of it. She began to cry and with a look of utter despair, I heard her say, 'Where's Shirley? I can't find Shirley.' Alzheimer's had stolen the essence of my Mom and who she once was. It was heartbreaking to watch and it still haunts me to this day."

-Sandy, (author's sister)
Daughter of Shirley who was diagnosed with
Alzheimer's disease at the age of 74.

There's a saying that goes, "Growing old is not for the faint of heart." Few of us would disagree especially if you are already in the throes of older age (depending on how you define it!) or have witnessed those ahead of you suffer from age-related debilitating conditions such as osteoarthritis, heart disease, high blood pressure, diabetes, or stroke. But one of the worst fears many of us share as years go by is losing our cognitive abilities. Staying physically in shape is important, but maintaining mental sharpness and acuity is just as vital. What a gift it is to be cognitively and socially active, participating fully in all aspects of life well into our elderly years.

Unfortunately, too many of us have been witness to loved ones taking a sharp decline when Alzheimer's disease or other forms of dementia take over. The person we once knew has vanished and been replaced with someone who we no longer recognize or often know how to interact with. Like a thief in the night, Alzheimer's disease quietly steals and wipes away a person's memory and life experiences.

What is Alzheimer's disease?

Alzheimer's disease is a chronic, irreversible, progressive brain disease, that slowly destroys memory and cognitive function. It is the most common cause of dementia. As of the writing of this book, for the year 2018, an estimated 5.7 million Americans of all ages are living with Alzheimer's dementia.

An in-depth look at the latest information from the Alzheimer's Association, *2018 Alzheimer's Disease Facts and Figures*,[1] gave a bleak forecast regarding the latest national statistics and information which was divided into three sections

1. Prevalence, Incidence, and Mortality:

- By 2025, the number of people age 65 and older with Alzheimer's dementia is estimated to reach 7.1 million - an increase of almost 29 percent from the 5.5 million age 65 and older affected in 2018.

- Unless there is a significant medical breakthrough, the number of people age 65 and older with Alzheimer's dementia may nearly triple from 5.5 million to 13.8 million by 2050. This is the population of New York City, Los Angeles, and Chicago combined.

- Two-thirds of Americans over age 65 with Alzheimer's dementia (3.4 million) are women.

- Every 65 seconds someone in the United States is given a diagnosis of Alzheimer's. By mid-century, someone in the U.S. will be diagnosed with the disease every 33 seconds.

- Alzheimer's is the sixth-leading cause of death in the U.S., and is the fifth-leading cause of death for those age 65 and older.

- As the population of the U.S. ages, Alzheimer's is becoming a more common cause of death, and it is the only top 10 causes of death that cannot be prevented, cured or even slowed.

2. Cost of Care:

- Total national cost of caring for those with Alzheimer's and other dementia is estimated at $277 billion (not including unpaid caregiving) in 2018, of which $186 billion is the cost to Medicare and Medicaid; out-of-pocket costs represent $60 billion of the total payments, while other costs total $30 billion.

- In 2017, the lifetime cost of care for a person living with dementia was $341,840 – with 70 percent of this cost borne by families directly through out-of-pocket costs and the value of unpaid care.

3. Caregiving:

- Nearly half of all caregivers (48 percent) who provide help to older adults do so for someone with Alzheimer's or another dementia.

- Approximately two-thirds of caregivers are women, and one-third of dementia caregivers are daughters.

- Forty-one percent of caregivers have a household income of $50,000 or less.

- It is estimated that the U.S. has approximately half the number of certified geriatricians that it currently needs, and only nine percent of nurse practitioners report having special expertise in gerontological care.

How Alzheimer's differs from other forms of dementia

While Alzheimer's accounts for 60 to 80 percent of dementia, it is not the only form. Many adults suffer from various types of dementia severe enough to interfere with their ability to live independently. Dementia is a general term for loss of memory that can also affect other mental abilities. Examples of other forms of dementia include the following:

- *Vascular dementia* – Second most common cause of dementia after Alzheimer's disease.

- *Dementia with Lewy bodies* – Lewy bodies are abnormal aggregations or clumps of the protein alpha-synuclein.

- *Mixed dementia* – More than one cause of dementia occurring simultaneously in the brain.

- *Parkinson's Disease* – As this disease progresses, it can result in a progressive dementia similar to dementia with Lewy bodies or Alzheimer's.

- *Normal Pressure Hydrocephalus* – Fluid builds up in the brain resulting in symptoms of difficulty walking, memory loss, and inability to control urination.

Individuals can have symptoms that mimic those of dementia without actually having it. Dementia-like symptoms can include depression, side effects from medications, thyroid problems, certain vitamin deficiencies and excessive use of alcohol. Unlike dementia, these conditions often may be reversed with treatment.

In 2012, the National Institute on Aging and Alzheimer's Association proposed new guidelines to help pathologists describe and categorize the brain changes associate with Alzheimer's disease.[2] In 2011, these two groups identified three stages of Alzheimer's. In the first stage, *preclinical Alzheimer's disease*, a person afflicted has no outward symptoms but does have some early brain changes detected through brain imaging and other biomarkers. In the second stage, *mild cognitive impairment*, a patient will exhibit very mild symptoms but can still perform everyday tasks. The third stage or *dementia due to Alzheimer's disease* is characterized by notable deficits in memory, thinking, and behavior affecting a patients' ability to function in daily life.

There is no single test proving a person has Alzheimer's disease. A diagnosis is made through a complete assessment considering all possible causes looking at medical history, physical exams, neurological exam, mental status tests, and brain imaging.

Because of the complexity of Alzheimer's disease, it is unlikely any one drug or other intervention can successfully treat it. Current approaches focus on helping people manage mental function and behavioral symptoms, as well as slowing or delaying the symptoms of the disease.

Many may not realize that dementia can even be caused by nutritional deficiencies such as pellagra, as a result of a deficiency of the B vitamin niacin, and hypocobalaminemia, a neurologic syndrome caused by a vitamin B12 deficiency.

Even if you never experience any form of dementia as you age, your brain is still vulnerable to cognitive changes known as mild cognitive impairment (MCI). Those with MCI – between 15 to 20 percent of elderly people - will have significant declines in their thinking, memory or reasoning abilities but will still be able to perform daily-life activities. It is possible they could go on to develop dementia but many with MCI never do.

Alzheimer's disease is a huge problem. Right now there are no drugs to stop the progress of this disease. If there is going to be any meaningful steps made toward slowing down or ideally preventing Alzheimer's altogether, it must be considered and addressed as a public health crisis.

All of us are aware of the significant ramifications of Alzheimer's and the tremendous effect it has on both the patient and the family. But yet, it doesn't seem to get quite the attention as other chronic illness such as cancer, heart disease, or diabetes. Maybe it's because Alzheimer's disease is hard to fathom or think about. In other words, it's scary.

We can be diagnosed with kidney disease that affects the kidneys or cancer that affects a certain organ of the body but rarely does anyone define themselves by that specific organ. Those diseases still leave a person mentally intact; it doesn't change our personhood or who we are. But cognitive decline is another story. We define ourselves by our thoughts, our feelings, and our intellect. Our cognitive ability is one of the most distinguishing features that separate human beings from all other species on earth. If our brain is affected by Alzheimer's, who are we then? What really goes on inside the mind of someone with this disease? None of us want to think about that.

But let's move away from the doom and gloom of the looming brain health crisis and focus on some good news. Never in the history of the human race, has the human life span been as long. More Americans are reaching the age of 100 than ever before.

In 2014, there were 72,197 Americans aged 100 or older, according to a report from the Centers for Disease Control and Prevention.[3] That number is up 44 percent from 2000, when there were only 50,281 centenarians.

Years ago, knowing someone who lived to be 100 was a rarity. Thanks to vast medical improvements over the decades – vaccines, antibiotics, safe drinking water, hygiene and sanitation, medications – the survival of people living longer and living well into old age has never been better.

But the increased length in years, also can take a toll on the body, depending on how well we take care of ourselves. Those of us living in the United States are far more likely to die as a result of a chronic disease such as cardiovascular disease, diabetes, hypertension, stroke, or cancer. However, Alzheimer's disease and other forms of dementia have joined the ranks as a leading cause of death as the number of elderly rises across the nation. In fact, the older one becomes, the greater likelihood that those who are physically fit enough to survive 100 years or more, will ultimately succumb to diseases afflicting the mind and cognitive dysfunction. Each passing year makes us more vulnerable to memory deficits and increased risk of dementia.

The challenge for the 21st Century will be to ensure that these added years are as healthy and productive as possible.

There is hope

As overwhelming and immense as the brain health crisis is, the one thing each of us can cling to is hope. Decades of dedicated researchers making it their life mission of finding new treatments to slow, stop, or preferably prevent Alzheimer's, thankfully continues. Though progress has been slow with many setbacks, minor successes have been made. Ultimately, we must never lose hope.

Hope is what spurs each of us to never give up the fight in finding a cure for this devastating disease. We should count our lucky stars for the visionaries who make it their life mission to strive to ultimately halt Alzheimer's destruction of the brain. Without these visionaries, there is no hope.

Fortunately, research is paving the way for providing clues to better understanding brain changes and brain health. Over the last 30 years, remarkable progress has been made in understanding the human brain and what happens as Alzheimer's develops.

There are drug therapies currently under investigation that show promise for future treatments or medications that would target certain areas of the brain:

- Beta-amyloid – A brain protein fragment, this sticky compound can accumulate in the brain, disrupting communication between brain cells and eventually killing them. This happens when beta-amyloid is broken from its parent compound amyloid precursor protein (APP) by two enzymes – beta-secretase and gamma-secretase. One goal of researchers is to develop medications that can block activity of these two enzymes thus preventing beta-amyloid fragments from clumping together into plaques.

- Tau proteins – A hallmark of Alzheimer's disease, tau protein perform the function of stabilizing microtubules and are a chief component of tangles, another common brain abnormality. Various strategies are being investigated to prevent tau proteins from collapsing and twisting into tangles, which destroys vital cell transport systems.

- Inflammation – A great deal has been learned about molecules involved in the body's overall inflammatory response. Inflammation is a key Alzheimer's abnormality and there is much interest in discovering and understanding inflammations effect on the brain. The hope is to develop innovative treatments for Alzheimer's disease that will reduce inflammation's damaging effect on brain health.

Keeping hope alive is key to combatting Alzheimer's disease.

Chapter Two

Understanding the Brain

"When my husband was no longer able to drive, I often took him on afternoon car rides, something he enjoyed. One day as we made our way to get in the car, he turned to me and said, 'Thank you for taking me for a ride, but just who are you?' Anger was my first instinct. Of course he knows who I am! That moment forced me to acknowledge the gravity of the extent of this disease. After being married for 56 years and raising two children, it was a heartbreaking realization I had to accept."

-Darlene
Wife and caretaker of her husband, Hummie
who was diagnosed with Alzheimer's disease
at the age of 79.

Interesting brain facts

Sitting on your shoulders is the most complicated organ known to medical science. This amazingly intricate part of the human body is astonishingly interesting yet few of us actually know much about it. Weighing about three pounds and composed of 75 percent water, your brain can identify what it's looking at approximately 30 times faster than you can blink your eye.

This rapid-fire processing was discovered by MIT neuroscientists who found that the human brain can process certain types of information within as little as 13 milliseconds[4]. To put that in perspective, it takes you 300 to 400 milliseconds to blink your eye, which is 1/3 of a second.

Even though your brain is primarily made up of water, remove the water and you're left with brain matter, 60 percent of which is fat, making it one of the fattest organs in the body. The fat found in the brain is an essential structural component of neurons of which there are astounding 100 billion present in this organ. These neurons or brain cells are irreplaceable. Cells in other parts of the body are constantly replaced when they die off. For example, skin cells and red blood cells replenish themselves about every 10 to 120 days, and cells lining the digestive tract die off and replace themselves every 3 days. But brain cells do not reproduce at all; if damaged by injury or disease, they are lost forever. This is why it is so important to pay attention to our brain health and the health of our brain cells.

Neurons have the amazing ability to gather and transmit electrochemical signals throughout the body. One neuron in the human brain may receive input from as many as one hundred thousand other neurons. The individual neurons form connections with other neurons by way of long, branching extensions. These connections allow information to flow in tiny bursts of chemicals released by one neuron and then detected by a receiving neuron. The synapses allow the signals to travel through the brain's neuronal circuits creating memories, thoughts, sensations, emotions, movements, and skills.

What is believed to contribute to the development of Alzheimer's disease is the accumulation of two substances – plaque and tau. Plaque is a protein beta-amyloid accumulating outside neurons. Tau, a protein produced naturally by healthy nerve cells, begins to form abnormally inside neurons. This abnormal version of tau accumulating during Alzheimer's disease prevents it from performing its job properly causing it to accumulate into *tau tangles*. When tau tangles accumulate, the number of synapses decline, information transfer at synapses fail and the neurons eventually die.

The plaque accumulation is believed to interfere with the neuron-to-neuron communication at the synapses. Tau tangles block the transport of nutrients and other essential molecules inside neurons. Accumulation of both plaque and tau tangles contribute to cell death resulting in dramatic brain shrinkage in people with advanced Alzheimer's.

Of course, we can't see our brain but did you know that you would be unable to tell if anything were actually touching it? This is a remarkable difference between the brain and the rest of our body. It is commonly believed that having a headache or migraine is due to pain generated inside the brain. That is not possible as there are no pain sensors in the brain. The *meninges* (coverings around the brain), periosteum (coverings on the bones), and the scalp all have pain receptors. If you were capable of touching your brain, you would not feel anything. This is why surgery can be performed on the brain, even while a patient is awake.

For instance, when you have a headache it may feel like a pain inside your brain, but it's not. Most headaches begin in the various nerves of the muscles and blood vessels surrounding your head, neck, and face. The nerves can sense pain set off by stress, muscle tension, enlarged blood vessels, and other triggers. Once activated, the nerves send messages to the brain, making it seem like the pain is coming from within your head.

Our hungry brain

The human brain also has a hungry appetite – even though it represents only two percent of your body weight it uses up to 20 percent of your daily calories, more than any other organ in the body. Every time you have a thought, make a move, or use any of your senses (sight, hearing, smell, touch, and taste), those 100 billion neurons are busy working. It takes a great deal of nutrients to keep your brain up and running every single second of each day.

Glucose, a type of sugar which is broken down from carbohydrates, is the preferred food and major fuel in the brain. It is transported across the cell membranes by a process called facilitated diffusion moderated by glucose transporter proteins. Our brain likes a steady supply of this sugar making it best to eat regular meals and snacks of healthy carbohydrate foods each day.

Antioxidants are another source of food our brain craves. An important reason our brain should have an ample supply of antioxidants is because of oxidative stress. Our body is under constant attack from oxidative stress which creates an imbalance from the production of free radicals. Every day every cell in the body makes thousands of free radicals which are unstable oxygen molecules. Our exposure to free radicals comes from various sources such as tobacco smoke, pollution, and even ultraviolet light. Left unchecked, free radicals scavenge the body causing damage to cells, proteins, DNA and have been associated with Alzheimer's disease.[5]

Antioxidants can come to the rescue by neutralizing free radicals preventing further damage. Think of antioxidants as the body's natural defense system to protect itself from oxidative stress. Antioxidants are supplied by well-known nutrients such as vitamins C and E, beta-carotene, and selenium. These vital nutrients help shield the body from the damage rogue free radicals can do.

As you can see, antioxidants do have their place in maintaining a healthy brain.

Inner workings of the brain

Now that you know how complex and fascinating your brain is, let's take an even more in-depth look at this organ. Surprisingly, the human brain is the most vulnerable organ in the body. For as vital and indispensable as it is, your brain needs the most protection of any organ. Anyone who has worked with cadavers and had the opportunity to actually hold a human brain in their hands will tell you how soft, mushy, and "jelly-like" it felt. Due to its high-fat content, it has a delicate texture making it easily susceptible to damage. It's no wonder nature encased our brain within the thick layers of our skull in addition to three layers of protective tissue called the meninges.

The term *meninges* comes from the Greek for "membrane" and refer to the three membranes that surround the brain and spinal cord. The membrane layers are the dura mater, arachnoid mater, and pia mater. The purpose of the meninges is to help anchor the central nervous system (CNS) in place to keep the brain from moving around within the skull. The meninges also contain cerebrospinal fluid which acts as a cushion for the brain and provides a solution in which the brain is suspended, allowing it to preserve its shape.

Your skull is a protective cavity for your brain. It helps to think of the skull as a virtual built-in helmet for your brain. This is why minor bumps to the head usually are not much to worry about. Even though your skull is a sturdy first line of defense, a much stronger, damaging major blow to the head can result in severe injury to the brain, if not death.

Within the skull is a clear, colorless liquid called cerebrospinal fluid. This liquid bathes the brain and spinal cord acting as a cushion for the brain within the skull and serves as a shock absorber for the central nervous system. Cerebrospinal fluid circulates nutrients and chemicals filtered from the blood and removes waste products from the brain keeping it clean and working up to par.

Between the skull, meninges, and cerebrospinal fluid, the brain is well-protected from external harm. But, nature also understood that your brain can come under assault from potentially harmful substances circulating in the bloodstream. To fight off any such antagonist possibly causing great harm, the brain is the only organ that has its own built-in security system – the *blood-brain barrier*.

The blood-brain barrier is a complex surrounding most of the blood vessels in the brain. It acts as a barrier between the bloodstream and the extracellular spaces of the brain allowing only certain substances like water, oxygen, nutrients, and small lipid-soluble substances to easily cross from the blood into the brain. This prevents toxins, pathogens, and other potentially dangerous substances from crossing the circulatory system into the brain.

It is thought that the central components of the structure of the blood-brain barrier are the tight junctions of the endothelial cells, the cells that make up the interior surface of blood vessels. In other blood vessels throughout the body there are small spaces between these endothelial cells. Small blood-borne substances can pass through these spaces and into surrounding tissues.

The endothelial cells that make up the blood-brain barrier however are tightly-fused together to form tight junctions that restrict diffusion across the blood vessel lining. This makes the barrier almost impermeable except for allowing only elements it recognizes as safe and necessary for coming in contact with the brain.

This high-security operation of how the blood-brain barrier works, gives the brain complete control over what is allowed to cross this barrier and what harmful substances are kept at bay.

Each day, all of us are bombarded by foreign particles wanting to do us and our brains harm. From bacteria, toxins, viruses, and even medications, the blood-brain barrier does its job of protecting the brain from infections and inflammation by restricting the passage of these antigens meaning to cause havoc.

After reading this chapter, you should have a much greater appreciation of your brain and just how extraordinarily amazing it is. The remaining chapters of this book explore the role of food and nutrition and what you need to know to properly nourish your brain to be as healthy as possible.

CHAPTER THREE

STUDIES ON FOOD'S ROLE IN BRAIN HEALTH

"We first realized something was seriously wrong with our Dad when he got up one night, walked across the street and knocked on his neighbor's door saying he couldn't find his house. Our worst fears were confirmed when his physician evaluated and diagnosed him with Alzheimer's disease. Eventually, the overwhelming caretaking duties were too much for Mom and the extraordinarily difficult decision was made to move him into a long-term care facility."

-Judy and George
Daughter-in-law and son of Harvey
who was diagnosed with Alzheimer's at age of 86

Science and food's role in brain health

The better you take care of your brain, the more fulfilling of a life you will have. This organ is so deeply tied to who you are as a person, to the world you live in, that brain health and doing what you can to avoid dementia and Alzheimer's, just makes good sense. One possibly promising strategy of reducing the onset of Alzheimer's may be your food choices.

In addition to aging, one of the strongest risk factors for the development and progression of cognitive decline and dementia is having a family history of it. Having relatives who developed Alzheimer's is out of our control, but one area we can be in charge of is our food choices.

We also know that there is a complex interaction between what we eat and how that can possibly reduce our risk of cognitive decline.

Our eating pattern encompasses what foods we choose from day to day, how often we eat certain foods, and in what quantity. Studies have shown that adopting certain dietary

patterns appear to have brain-protecting qualities each of us should embrace. This chapter will focus primarily on the MIND diet which may have substantial benefits for the prevention of Alzheimer's disease.

The MIND Diet

In the world of nutrition, every so often a study comes out making you stop and think about the real-life applications that could possibly benefit so many people. In March 2015, a study heralding a pattern of eating was published in *Alzheimer's & Dementia: The Journal of the Alzheimer's Association* that not only made headline news but showed much promise of making a dent in the growing tally of individuals diagnosed with Alzheimer's.[6] The findings and applications from this study are still reverberating around the world.

A nutritional epidemiologist at Rush University Medical Center, Martha Clare Morris, PhD, developed the MIND diet that may significantly lower a person's risk of developing Alzheimer's disease.

Supporting this theory are results from two randomized trials showing that dietary patterns influence cognitive decline. The first trial in 2013 found that after 6.5 years of following the Mediterranean diet, individuals had significantly higher scores on the Mini-Mental State Examination (MMSE) and Clock Drawing Test compared with the control diet participants.[7] The second trial participants on the Dietary Approaches to Stop Hypertension (DASH) diet had better improvements compared with the control diet.[8]

The encouraging findings from this research were that older adults who adhered to a DASH and Mediterranean diet pattern, experienced slower rates of cognitive decline. This information spurred the development of a new diet, essentially a hybrid of the Mediterranean and DASH diets, designed to protect the brain called the Mediterranean-DASH diet Intervention for Neurodegenerative Delay (MIND).[9] Both diets are intertwined but with modifications based on findings of studies looking at using diet to delay or prevent dementia. The objective was to relate the MIND diet score to cognitive decline in the Memory and Aging Project (MAP) and to compare the estimated effects to those of the Mediterranean and DASH diets that were found to be protective against cognitive decline among the MAP study participants.[10]

The Mediterranean diet is culturally based in Mediterranean countries (e.g., Greece, Turkey, Lebanon) and emphasizes the cooking style of that region. This eating pattern is comprised of mainly whole, minimally-processed plant foods including cereal grains, legumes, vegetables, fruit and nuts, fish, small amounts of meat, milk, and dairy products and a regular modest amount of alcohol, such as red wine.[11] It's been shown to be beneficial for heart health by lowering the risk of heart attack, stroke, high blood pressure, and high blood cholesterol.[7]

The DASH diet emphasizes fruit, vegetables, and low-fat dairy products as well as whole grains, poultry, fish, and nuts, and is reduced in fats, red meat, sweets, and sugar-containing beverages.[11] The primary focus of this eating pattern, more so than the Mediterranean diet, is to lower high blood pressure. It encourages reduction of sodium while recommending an increased intake of foods that are good sources of the minerals potassium, calcium, and magnesium to lower high blood pressure.

By combining the Mediterranean and DASH diets, the MIND diet emphasizes natural, plant-based foods, promotes an increase in the consumption of berries and green leafy vegetables, and limits intake of animal protein and foods high in saturated fats. There are 15 dietary components of the MIND diet.[12] Ten components are the "brain-healthy" foods and the other five components are listed under "unhealthy."

10 Brain-Healthy Foods

1	**Green leafy vegetables**	At least six servings a week (spinach, kale, romaine, etc)
2	**Other vegetables**	At least one serving a day
3	**Nuts**	At least five servings a week
4	**Berries**	At least two or more servings a week
5	**Beans**	At least three servings a week
6	**Whole grains**	At least three or more servings a day
7	**Fish**	At least once a week
8	**Poultry**	At least two times a week (chicken or turkey)
9	**Olive oil**	Used as your main oil
10	**Wine**	One glass a day (5 ounces)

	5 Unhealthy Foods	
1	**Red meat**	Less than four servings a week choosing lean cuts (round or sirloin and graded "choice" or "select" instead of "prime" which has more fat)
2	**Butter or margarine**	Less than a tablespoon a day
3	**Cheese**	Less than one serving a week
4	**Pastries and sweets**	Less than five servings a week
5	**Fried or fast food**	Less than one serving a week

Notice that berries are the only fruit mentioned in the MIND diet. Other fruits can certainly be used but berries are singled out due to their formidable power in keeping the brain healthy. Blueberries in particular contain a compound called anthocyanins, a pigment and powerful compound which may help boost cognitive function.

Anthocyanins is found in many plant-based foods, especially in blueberries and strawberries, as they provide the bright blue and red colors of these fruits. Past studies have shown the neurological improvements blueberries provide due to anthocyanins that seem to reduce oxidative stress, decreases inflammation, and increase signaling between neurons.[13]

How the MIND diet works

The good thing about the MIND diet is how it can be easily applied to other forms of dementia besides Alzheimer's. *Vascular dementia*, which is the second most common form of dementia caused by reduced blood flow to the brain usually from a stroke or series of strokes, is one such example of this. In 2012, a study looked at nutrition as one of the main modifiable variables that may influence the development of it.[14] Results from the study found specific nutritional components support vascular health which in turn can protect against vascular dementia. Those nutritional components from the study included antioxidants, lipids, homocysteine, folate, and vitamin B12, all nutrients found in abundance in the MIND diet.

There were a couple of nutrients in particular strongly associated with the MIND diet – vitamin E and the omega-3 fatty acid, docosahexaenoic acid or DHA. Vitamin E, found in nuts, plant oils, seeds, and leafy greens has a strong association for improving brain health. Another food encouraged by the MIND diet is fish, an excellent source of omega-3 fatty acids. In the brain, omega-3's are important for synaptic proteins which lead to higher synaptic transmission and less oxidative stress in addition to being an important part of lipid structure. The B vitamin folate along with vitamins C and D have also been found to help neurons cope with aging.[15]

Food choices may possibly make a significant difference whether a person may possibly develop Alzheimer's or not. The emphasis of certain foods associated with the MIND diet appears to demonstrate this. Even though the MIND diet emphasizes natural plant-based foods and limits intake of animal protein and foods high in saturated fat, the unique emphasis of consuming berries and green leafy vegetables sets it apart. The MIND diet does not emphasize a high consumption of fruit (both Mediterranean and DASH do), dairy (DASH does), or eating more fish each week (Mediterranean). The MIND diet instead shines a spotlight on the foods and nutrients associated with dementia prevention based on scientific literature.

Many individuals, including medical professionals, often believe loss of cognitive functioning is simply an accepted and almost expected natural consequence of aging. This belief was also common during the mid-20th century of the perception of heart failure. At that time, scientists and doctors understood the heart's physiology and its potential for failure, but an understanding of the association between heart failure and a person's lifestyle and food choices was missing.

Decades of research has shown how healthful dietary and lifestyle choices, when started early in life and continued through one's lifespan, have a profoundly positive effect on maintaining heart health and increased life expectancy.

Today, research is linking together those same components of keeping our heart strong and healthy – good nutrition and lifestyle choices – to keeping our brain healthy and functioning at its best well into old age.

PART 2
BRAIN-HEALTHY NOURISHMENT

CHAPTER FOUR
_____

ESSENTIAL NUTRIENTS FOR THE BRAIN

"Looking back on my Dad's battle with Alzheimer's, I realize how many of the things he enjoyed in life were taken from him in the disease process. For example, he began to decline invitations from friends to play cards or dominoes. We thought this was unusual since Dad was always a social person. Later, we discovered he just couldn't understand rules to games anymore and didn't want to tell anyone. Watching sporting events had been a favorite of his, but on one outing to watch a granddaughter play softball, he leaned over and asked me, 'What are they doing out there?' Something so familiar to him had become meaningless. Any moments of clarity for my Dad were fleeting and something our family cherished as the disease progressed."

-Marla
Daughter of Dean, who was diagnosed
with Alzheimer's disease at the age of 71

A lifetime of nutrient nourishment

There is not enough that can be said of the overall impact of food choices on a person's health during their lifetime. Each day, you make numerous decisions on what foods you are going to eat. Depending on the nutrient composition of the food you eat, its nutritional value will likely have cumulative effects on your body, including your brain. Basically, whatever foods you choose day-to-day, determines the nutrients you are feeding your body.

Most individuals are familiar with the term "nutrient" but may be unsure exactly what a nutrient is. Nutrients are components found within food that are necessary for the body to function properly. Nutrients are what provide us with energy. Nutrients fuel your body to stay alert all day at work. Nutrients provide you with energy to workout at the gym for 30 minutes or more. Nutrients help us grow from infancy to adulthood. Nutrients help maintain or repair body tissue necessary for healing wounds. When you are lacking sufficient nutrients, you will notice the effects such as feeling sluggish or having a weakened immune system.

The human body requires six different kinds of nutrients: Carbohydrates, protein, fat, vitamins, minerals and water.

The first three - carbohydrates, protein, and fat - are also known as the "energy-yielding" or "calorie-yielding nutrients", meaning they supply your body energy or calories (in the world of nutrition these terms are synonymous). These three nutrients are also called *macronutrients* meaning they are necessary in large amounts for the human body. Every single bite of food we eat, whether it's a grilled cheese sandwich or a green salad, contains a proportion or combination of different macronutrients. Much of your foods are composed of a combination of all three macronutrients. A hamburger on a bun, for example, would be a combination of carbohydrates, protein, and fat. However, some foods such as oils (e.g., olive or canola) are composed of one hundred percent oil whereas a teaspoon of granulated sugar is one hundred percent carbohydrate. Each of the macronutrients not only supply energy but also have various other functions in the body from providing materials that form structures of body tissue to helping absorb other nutrients from our food.

Vitamins and minerals are referred to as *micronutrients* as they are needed by your body in only trace amounts – in other words, the body doesn't require much of them in order to do their work.

Micronutrients do not provide the body with energy or calories. Their main function is to act as regulators. As regulators, vitamins and minerals assist and are heavily involved in every process necessary to maintain life: digesting food, moving muscles, disposing wastes, growing new tissues, healing wounds, and extracting energy from carbohydrates, fat, and protein.

The sixth nutrient – water - like vitamins and minerals, also does not provide calories but is crucial for us just to remain alive. Water has numerous functions in our body such as acting as a lubricant, cleansing the blood of waste, and transporting nutrients to regulate body temperature. Most of us could survive several weeks without food but it'd be only a matter of a few days without water before you would succumb to death. Your body does not make or store water. Whatever water you lose daily from sweating, urinating, or respiration, must be replaced by either drinking it or from other fluids and food sources containing it.

Ideally each of us would choose to eat a majority of foods high in nutrient density. Nutrient density is a measure of nutrients provided per calorie of food. In other words, a nutrient-dense food provides vitamins, minerals, and other beneficial substances with relatively few calories. For example, if you wanted to increase your calcium intake, a couple of food choices that both supply this mineral would be ice cream and one percent low-fat milk. If you chose a cup of rich ice cream containing more than 350 calories instead of a cup of one percent low-fat milk which has only 100 calories and almost double the calcium, it's clear which one is more nutrient dense.

Next, let's take a closer look at specific nutrients that have been found appearing to play a special role in maintaining brain health.

B Vitamins and Brain Health

There has been significant research in the role B vitamins play in maintaining cognitive function.[16] Even though we may not be totally able to prevent age-related cognitive declines, the B vitamins seem to have an edge in perhaps doing so.

There are eight B vitamins which include thiamine (B1), riboflavin (B2), niacin (B3), pantothenic acid (B5), vitamin B6, also known as pyridoxine, biotin (B7), folate (B9), and vitamin B12. Each B vitamin has jobs related to cognitive function as each is transported across the blood-brain barrier with active roles in making brain chemicals called neurotransmitters helping to communicate information.

ESSENTIAL NUTRIENTS FOR THE BRAIN

Another factor in keeping our brain healthy revolves around an amino acid called *homocysteine*. The B vitamins keep homocysteine levels in a healthy range.

In particular adequate intake of vitamin B12 is required for the methylation of homocysteine meaning it adds a methyl group to this amino acid – Methyl groups are a common structural unit of organic compounds consisting of three hydrogen atoms bonded to a carbon atom, which is linked to the remainder of the molecule. If you were to consume less than what is recommended of vitamin B12, this increases levels of homocysteine leaving the brain not as well protected.

High homocysteine levels have been linked with a greater risk of age-related cognitive decline, brain shrinkage, and an increased risk of Alzheimer's disease.[17] Vitamin B12 is found naturally only in foods of animal origin (e.g., beef, pork, lamb, poultry, fish, eggs, milk and milk products). Therefore, meeting vitamin B12 needs is a concern among vegans – those who consume no animal products. In order to prevent the scenario of low vitamin B12 and high homocysteine levels, vegans, must take a vitamin B12 supplement or consume foods fortified with the vitamin such as fortified breakfast cereals or soymilk.

Since absorption of vitamin B12 is often reduced in older adults, the National Institutes of Health recommends all adults older than age 50 to take vitamin B12 supplements.[18]

The B vitamin folate has as a role in energy production in the brain and aids in the production of DNA and RNA – the body's genetic material.

An interesting function of folate that may possibly be related to brain health is that it increases nitric oxide, which protects the arterial endothelium. When nitric oxide is widely available, this improves *vasoconstriction* and *vasodilation* which is the narrowing and widening of blood vessels that control blood flow. It is known that one key to preventing heart disease and stroke is to protect the endothelium from oxidative damage. But it is not entirely understood if this same protection applies to protecting the brain and cognitive function. One study has shown that older adults who consumed adequate foods high in folate had the lowest rates of Alzheimer's.[19]

Another study found that individuals who did not consume adequate levels of folate led to an increase in serum homocysteine which researchers associate with reduced cognitive function in old age.[20] This has been called the *homocysteine hypothesis*.

An inadequate intake of folate can also inhibit repair of DNA while increasing the susceptibility of oxidative damage to the brain's neurons. Eventually, this could begin the setup towards developing cognitive decline.

The recommended intake of folate for adults is 400 micrograms (mcg) a day, Researchers in the Netherlands gave 800 participants, all who had low folate intake and elevated homocysteine at baseline, either 800 mcg of folic acid a day or a placebo for three years.[21]

At the end of the three years, those who received the 800 mcg of folic acid a day, scored higher on memory and cognition tests than those who received the placebo. Before anyone decides to start taking a folic acid supplement for brain health, it is recommended to use food sources of folate first. Anyone taking a folic acid supplement needs to follow-up with their physician as excess folate intake can mask a vitamin B12 deficiency.

Vitamin E and Brain Health

Unlike the B vitamins which are called "water-soluble vitamins," vitamin E is one of four vitamins (the other three are A, D, & K), that are called "fat-soluble vitamins". The fat-soluble vitamins are found in the fats and oils of foods and require bile and fat for absorption. Once absorbed, these vitamins are stored in the liver and fatty tissues until the body needs them.

There are four forms of vitamin E – alpha tocopherol, beta tocopherol, delta tocopherol, and gamma tocopherol. Alpha tocopherol (the only form found in vitamin supplements) and gamma tocopherol both have anti-inflammatory and antioxidant properties.

Vitamin E is an antioxidant. Think of antioxidants as a bodyguard protecting against oxidative damage. This type of damage can occur when highly unstable molecules known as free radicals are formed during normal cell metabolism. If free radicals were left unchecked, they would wreak havoc throughout the body causing destructive damage to DNA in genetic material and disrupting the process of how proteins work within cells.

The good news is your body has the built-in natural defense of antioxidants from both nutrients and enzyme to fight off free radicals. This is why nutrients like vitamin E are imperative to fighting with free radicals and helping protect and preserve the health of your body. This also makes it necessary to do what you can to replenish these antioxidants daily by making smart food choices.

Being an antioxidant, gives vitamin E certain functions essential for good health such as strengthening the immune system, forming red blood cells, and helping the body use vitamin K.

Due to its antioxidant behavior, vitamin E has shown to be viable for brain health. It helps to protect the brain from oxidative stress and thwart potential damage to neural tissue within the brain. If one becomes deficient in this nutrient, several symptoms related to declining brain health appear including cognitive decline, loss of control over bodily movements, reduced reflex ability, and paralyzed eye muscles.

Unfortunately, when compared to other body organs, the brain has few antioxidant nutrients and enzymes. Vitamin E however, lives within the neuron cell membranes making it an important antioxidant for the brain. Vitamin E attacks free radicals and prevents them from disrupting and damaging brain cells. Studies have shown vitamin E uses its antioxidant and anti-inflammatory powers to protect neurons from oxidative damage and the development of amyloid plaques of Alzheimer's disease.[22] These same studies have also found vitamin E plays a role in preserving memory, cognitive function, and possibly reducing the risk of Alzheimer's disease.

Carotenoids and Flavonoids and Brain Health

Within plant-based foods are substances called *carotenoids* and *flavonoids*. Both are considered to be phytonutrients or plant chemicals and both have various health-promoting qualities.

Carotenoids are plant pigments responsible for the red, orange, and deep yellow colors found in many fruits and vegetables. There are more than 600 carotenoids found in nature, but only about 50 are found in the typical human diet. These special phytonutrients help plants absorb light energy for use in photosynthesis. The five most common carotenoids are alpha-carotene, beta-carotene, lutein, lycopene, and zeaxanthin.

Flavonoids are a diverse group of phytonutrients and are found in almost all fruits and vegetables. They also provide the vivid colors in produce. There are more than 6,000 types of flavonoids making them the largest group of phytonutrients with one of the best known being quercetin.

Phytonutrients such as carotenoids and flavonoids have only recently been found to contain powerful antioxidants with anti-inflammatory and immune system benefits.

Research has also found in recent years that the carotenoids, lutein and zeaxanthin, may be useful in maintaining cognitive function in the elderly. Data from various studies have supported the importance of these two carotenoids in brain health.[23] Lutein is the predominant carotenoid in the brain and is absorbed by the brain more than any other carotenoid.

Years of oxidative stress and inflammation can make the brain vulnerable to decreases in cognitive functioning. What may help are dietary antioxidants and anti-inflammatory agents that delay oxidative damage to the brain. Lutein and zeaxanthin function both as an antioxidant and anti-inflammatory agents in order to maintain proper brain functioning.

One study of healthy, older women who received 12 milligrams of lutein along with 800 milligrams of DHA (an omega-3 fatty acid) per day were found to have improved verbal fluency, memory scores, and a higher learning rate after 4 months.[24] Studies such as this help support the role of carotenoids in improving brain health like lutein and zeaxanthin working together synergistically with DNA.

Flavonoid research and brain health is not as extensive as carotenoid research and have mainly been done on animal studies rather than human studies. But of the studies that have been conducted, they have consistently shown flavonoids to have positive benefits for reducing cognitive decline and possible reduction of inflammation of neurons in the brain.[25]

Dietary fat and brain health

Few people question the health benefits of fruits and vegetables or other plant-based foods, but when it comes to fat in the diet, many are confused and conflicted over their fat choices.

What you need to know is there are three types of fat in the human diet: monounsaturated, polyunsaturated, and saturated. The major distinction between these three is that saturated fat is usually solid at room temperature (i.e., butter, stick margarine, fat found in meat) while mono- and polyunsaturated fats are usually liquid at room temperature (e.g.., canola, corn, or olive oil).

If you consume a diet rich in saturated fats, this can increase your risk for developing cardiovascular disease. However, choosing foods rich in mono- and polyunsaturated fats, helps reduce atherosclerosis and the risk of heart disease and stroke.

The overall goal for anyone in their approach to fat consumption is to choose more mono- and polyunsaturated fats than saturated fat. But be mindful of the fact that anytime fat is lowered in a food product, food manufacturers likely increased the sugar content substantially to make it palatable. A food label stating "no fat" or "low fat" most likely has a higher sugar content. If it didn't, the food would not as appetizing since most of the fat was removed. A high sugar intake is also not advisable as sugar has little to no nutritional value even though scientific evidence is lacking on its effect on brain health.

Individuals who eat a lot of foods high in saturated fat such as pizza, cheese, red meat, and high-fat dairy, have about double the risk for developing Alzheimer's disease.[26] These same people eating high saturated fat diets were also shown in another study that when compared with individuals who had a high consumption of polyunsaturated and monounsaturated fat, those eating more saturated fats suffered a more significant decline in their cognitive abilities.[27]

Omega-3 fatty acids are another type of fat well-known for its role in heart health. Today, more evidence is supporting its use in protecting your brain. Omega-3 fatty acids are a type of polyunsaturated fat that is divided into three groups – DHA, EPA, and ALA. Eicosapentaenoic acid (EPA) and docosahexaenoic acid (DHA) are found mainly in fish and are sometimes called marine omega-3s. Alpha-linolenic acid (ALA) is the most common omega-3 fatty acid in most Western diets, and is found in vegetable oils and nuts (especially walnuts), flax seeds and flaxseed oil, leafy vegetables and some animal fat, especially grass-fed animals. The human body generally uses ALA for energy, and conversion into EPA and DHA is very limited. While the human body can make most of the types of fats it needs from other fats or raw materials, this isn't the case for omega-3 fatty acids. Omega-3 fatty acids are essential fats because the body can't make them and we must get them from food.

Much research has shown that omega-3 fatty acids are vital to the brain and normal brain function. They have been shown to be instrumental in neurocognitive development starting in utero and continuing through the early childhood years.

Remember that the brain is predominately composed of fat of which DHA is the primary brain lipid (fat). The cerebral cortex, the synaptic terminals, and the mitochondria are the most metabolically active areas of the brain of which DNA is particularly abundant. As you age, your DHA levels decrease due to oxidative stress. To reduce this natural progression, it would be advisable to consume more of the best sources of DHA which are fatty fish such as salmon, tuna, sardines, mackerel, or herring.

CHAPTER FIVE

FOOD FOR THOUGHT – BRAIN-SUSTAINING AND BRAIN-DRAINING FOODS

"When my wife was diagnosed with Alzheimer's, it was only a short matter of time before I saw significant changes. It was not unusual for her to wake up shortly past midnight, one or two o'clock, packing her bags stating she had had enough and was leaving me. It would take several hours to calm her down and when morning arrived, she had no recollection of the previous night. Throughout our marriage she was well-known for her talent with crafts and scrapbooking but those hobbies no longer held interest for her. A once vibrant and engaging person, towards the end, I would often catch her staring straight ahead, her eyes showing nothing."

-Dennis
Husband and caretaker of his wife, Jean who was
diagnosed with Alzheimer's disease at the age of 67.

Whether you pay much attention to your food choices or not, let me say this: you should. Obviously, this book is addressing foods for optimizing your brain health as best you can. But healthy eating simply makes sense in all areas of health such as cardiovascular, kidney, bone, skin, and muscle mass. This will likely enhance the number of years you will live but more importantly, enhance the quality of those years bringing you more fulfillment, energy, and joy.

Your overall eating pattern encompasses what foods you choose every day, how often you eat certain foods and in what quantities. From what I have presented in this book so far, adopting a dietary pattern mimicking a Mediterranean-style diet or a more plant-based diet is what appears to be the most brain-protecting eating pattern around.

The Mediterranean diet is a term used to describe the traditional eating habits of people living in Greece, Italy, and other Mediterranean countries. The dietary pattern includes nutrient-rich, plant-based foods like leafy green vegetables, berries, and extra-virgin olive oil.

Healthy eating patterns such as the Mediterranean diet help promote better blood sugar which could help protect brain function as cognitive decline has been observed in older people who have impaired glucose tolerance. It is known that having insulin sensitivity and diabetes are risk factors for dementia. Any diet that is largely made up of sugar and refined grains has the risk of increasing cognitive decline.

Brain-Sustaining Foods

Chapters three and four covered the science behind the role nutrients within our food provide for brain health and reducing risk of Alzheimer's and dementia. This chapter takes a look at specific foods best to include in a brain-healthy diet.

To preserve and enhance brain health, your food choices should be filled with brain-optimizing nutrients. To help you discover what specific foods are best for your brain, it helps to categorize foods into food groups.

Valuable Vegetables

Vegetables are a true asset nature provides us for getting and keeping you healthy. One of the best ways to get to know your vegetables is to spend a little more time in the produce section at your grocery store. Many of you may always buy the same vegetables time and time again without realizing the vast array and options you have to choose from.

When making those decisions, look for two things in particular – the color green and leafy. Leafy dark green vegetables are our ally in protecting cognitive abilities as we age. Chock-full of brain-enhancing nutrients such as folate, lutein, vitamin E, and beta-carotene, these veggies are your top powerhouse produce for keeping your brain functioning at its best.

I want to emphasize that the darker the leaves in leafy green vegetables, the greater source of brain-healthy nutrients. Pale Iceberg lettuce can be enjoyed as the foundation for salads, however, it is not considered a "dark" leafy green. The intense dark green color signals the abundance of the plant pigment carotenoids and other polyphenolic compounds that will nourish your thinking skills.

To help slow cognitive decline, the recommended consumption of a dark leafy green is at least one serving a day. Here is a listing of the best of dark leafy greens for you to choose from:

- Arugula
- Broccoli
- Collard greens
- Kale
- Mustard greens
- Spinach
- Swiss chard
- Turnip greens

Since some of the nutrients in dark leafy greens are fat soluble, these will be best absorbed if healthy oil is used as a dressing. You can make your own healthy salad dressing by simply mixing 2 tablespoons of extra-virgin olive oil with a teaspoon of both lemon juice and red-wine vinegar.

The dark leafy greens listed above are usually eaten raw within a salad. However, don't overlook cooking these same vegetables to unlock even more of their nutrient potential. For example, spinach which most of us consume raw, contains oxalic acid, that blocks the absorption of calcium and iron, two important nutrients for good health. Briefly heating spinach to a high temperature will break down oxalic acid. Simply cook spinach in boiling water for one minute, then plunge in ice water for a few minutes. Drain the spinach well and keep in an airtight-container in the refrigerator to be used in salads.

Many of the same dark leafy greens can be thrown into a stir fry, soup, or smoothie for anyone who wants to "hide" their bitter flavors.

Besides dark leafy greens, many other vegetables are also valuable for their nutrient contribution for good cognitive functioning. Each day, aim to have at least two types of nutrient-dense veggies that also offer a slew of important nutrients to protect your brain health:

- Asparagus
- Beets
- Brussel sprouts
- Cabbage
- Carrots
- Cauliflower
- Celery
- Cucumber
- Eggplant
- Green beans
- Leeks
- Mushrooms
- Okra
- Onions
- Peas
- Pumpkins
- Radishes
- Squash
- Sweet peppers
- Sweet potatoes
- Zucchini

As mentioned previously, how you prepare your vegetables makes a difference on the amount of nutrients your body is absorbing. Fat-soluble vitamins like vitamin E and carotenoids are enhanced rather than reduced when cooked.

To gain the most nutritional value, your best bet is to consume a variety of both raw and cooked vegetables.

No matter whether you like your vegetables fresh, frozen, or canned, all are similar in their nutritional content so you can feel confident in whichever method you prefer and can afford. Of course, the most nutritious option would be picking a vegetable straight from the garden at its peak ripeness and eating it right away. But the majority of us do not have that luxury. It is true that the nutritional content of fresh vegetables depends on various factors, including seasonality and availability. Many of the vegetables in grocery stores have traveled a long distance and may have been exposed to extreme light and temperature differences, all of which can cause a loss of important nutrients such as thiamine and vitamins A and C. Farmer's markets are a good option for vegetables grown locally and picked at their nutritional peak.

Frozen vegetables are always an excellent choice for providing the same essential nutrients and health benefits as fresh produce. Frozen vegetables are just like fresh but have been blanched (cooked for a short time in boiling water or steamed) and then frozen within hours after being harvested. They also are processed at their peak in terms of freshness and nutrition.

Canned vegetables can be a good option but the canning process does affect nutritional content such as loss of vitamin C in the high-heat temperature used for canning. These vegetables are also picked at peak ripeness, blanched and then canned. A caveat of canned vegetables is that sodium is added to preserve flavor and prevent spoilage. If excess sodium is a concern, choose "No-Salt Added" versions of canned vegetables instead or after opening the can, drain contents into a colander and rinse well under cold running water up to a minute to reduce the sodium content up to 40 percent.

Aim for 5 servings of vegetables each day with a serving considered as either 1 cup raw or ½ cup cooked.

Favored Fruits

A favorite food group of mine, fruit practically brims with health-promoting nutrients good for feeding your body and brain. Packed with antioxidants and phytochemicals, it's hard to go wrong with fruit. Just a quick rinse and it's ready-to-go. Delicious and nutritious, fruit lends itself to be easily added to hot or cold cereals, yogurt, salads, or liquefied into a smoothie.

But, when it comes to the biggest brain boost, berries rise to the top. The small but mighty berry is quite powerful in its approach to fighting cognitive decline. Its brain-healthy superpowers come from carotenoids and flavonoids, the phytochemicals possessing antioxidant and anti-inflammatory properties.

One fruit especially rich in the flavonoid anthocyanin, blueberries are packed with this antioxidant to support brain health increasing cognitive abilities. In animal studies, anthocyanins have promising implications for Alzheimer's disease by possibly improving memory function through growth of neurons in the brain's memory region.

A daily handful of blueberries are a recommended way to keep your brain healthy. Regular consumption of blueberries may be one strategy to forestall or even reverse age-related neuronal deficits. The polyphenolic compounds found in this sweet berry also help lower oxidative stress and inflammation by destroying free radicals that cause damage at the cellular level of all organs including brain cells.

Research on older adults who were given 1 cup of blueberries (powdered) for 90 days, showed improvement at remembering what they had already said when compared to those who were given a placebo.[28] They also showed improved accuracy when switching between tasks. This is believed to be attributed to the colorful phytochemical anthocyanin which may help control oxidative damage and inflammation in the brain.

Blueberries are not the only berry to rely on for boosting brain health. Choosing a variety of berries throughout the week is perfect for obtaining the brain-enhancing compounds each contains. Here is a list of nutrient-dense berries keeping your brain sharp:

- Acai berries
- Blackberries
- Blueberries
- Cranberries
- Raspberries
- Strawberries

Aim for 4 servings of fruit a day. A serving of fresh, frozen or canned fruit is the size of a tennis ball; a serving of dried fruit or fruit juice is ¼ cup.

Whole Grains and Brain Health

Misconceived as being a drain on brain health, whole grains are an important part of protecting your brain thanks to rich source of B vitamins and moderate amounts of vitamin E.

Before going any further, it is necessary to define what the term "whole grain" means.

Whole grains offer a "complete package" of health benefits. Unlike refined grains, which are stripped of valuable nutrients in the refining process, whole grains (wheat, corn, barley, rye, rice) contain three parts: bran, germ, and endosperm. Each of these parts house health-promoting nutrients. The bran is the hard outer layer and is rich in fiber, B vitamins, several minerals, protein, and phytochemicals. The germ is the core of the seed where growth occurs and is rich in healthy fats, vitamin E, B vitamins, phytochemicals, and antioxidants. The endosperm is the interior layer that contains starch, protein, and some vitamins and minerals.

When you see the word "refined" on an ingredient list, it means the bran and germ layers were removed during the milling process, leaving just the starchy endosperm. Milling is the process of crushing and grinding a whole grain to produce flour. When the brain and germ have been removed, this means there is significant loss of soluble and insoluble fiber, B vitamins, minerals including calcium, iron, and magnesium, and antioxidant compounds. Basically, milling whole wheat into refined wheat flour such as white flour strips away 70 to 80 percent of its vitamins and antioxidants.

There is actually scant research on whole grains effect on cognition and dementia. But whole grains and the fiber they contain have been shown to reduce the risk of developing cardiovascular risk factors that can lead to issues with cognition – hypertension, diabetes, obesity, and coronary heart disease.

For those who must avoid gluten (a protein found only in wheat, barley, and rye) due to celiac disease or have non-celiac gluten sensitivity (also called "gluten sensitivity"), there are whole grain alternatives which include amaranth, buckwheat, corn, millet, quinoa, rice, sorghum, and teff.

Here is a list of nutrient-dense whole grains to include in your daily diet:

- Amaranth
- Barley
- Buckwheat
- Brown and wild rice
- Bulgur
- Corn
- Farro aka Emmer
- Freekeh
- Kamut berries
- Kaniwa
- Millet
- Oats
- Popcorn
- Quinoa
- Rye
- Sorghum
- Spelt
- Teff
- Triticale
- Wheat berries

The Dietary Guidelines for Americans recommends that all adults eat at least half of their grains as whole grains or to have between 3 to 5 servings a day of whole grains. Here are examples of what one serving of whole grains is equivalent to:

- ½ cup cooked brown rice or other cooked grain
- ½ cup cooked 100% whole-grain pasta
- ½ cup cooked hot cereals, such as oatmeal
- 1 ounce uncooked whole-grain pasta, brown rice or grain
- 1 slice 100% whole wheat bread
- 1 ounce serving of 100% whole-grain muffin
- 1 cup 100% whole-grain ready-to-eat cereal

Brain-Nourishing Nuts

It's hard to go wrong with nuts. Portable, no cooking required, can be kept at room temperature, an easy snack - nuts are also an excellent brain-healthy food.

Ever so popular, nuts are well-known for having a heart healthy nutritional punch but now we know nuts also give our brain a boost. Thanks to their omega-3 fatty acids content, nuts are necessary for neuron growth and plasticity possibly fighting against age-related changes. Your body does not make omega-3 fatty acids so they must be obtained from your diet.

Years ago, nuts were shunned as being "too rich in fat." Today that thought has changed and nuts are no longer snubbed as being unhealthy. Nuts are some of the healthiest and best sources of both monounsaturated and polyunsaturated fats which also appear to support brain heath. A study called the PREDIMED clinical trial found improvements in memory of older adults who were given about one ounce of mixed nuts daily to eat as part of a Mediterranean diet for 4 years compared to older adults who ate a normal diet.[29]

There are many nuts to choose from but if you had to pick one that stands head-and-shoulders above the rest in regards to brain enhancement, walnuts would be the winner.

Walnuts have been studied extensively and are associated with better memory scores and cognitive function.[30]

What makes walnuts special is they are one of the nuts highest in gamma tocopherol and have the highest composition of polyunsaturated fatty acids, including alpha linoleic acid. Studies looking at walnut consumption believe it is the high polyphenol (antioxidants) present in walnuts that may help counteract age-related cognitive decline and reduce the incidence of neurodegenerative diseases, including Alzheimer's disease.[31]

To maximize the most from nuts and their brain-boosting abilities, eat about 1 ounce – roughly a small handful or about ¼ of a cup– of a variety of nuts at least 4-5 times a week if not daily. Nuts are good for us but nuts also are high in calories – be careful as overindulging could lead to weight gain. As healthy as walnuts and other nuts can be, 1 ounce or ¼ cup of almonds has 160 calories and 1 ounce or ¼ cup of walnuts has 210 calories. Eat much more than 1 ounce and the calories quickly add up!

The nice thing about nuts is their versatility. They can be easily tossed onto a salad or stir-fry, blended into a smoothie or mixed with brown rice, yogurt, or hot oatmeal for added crunch. It's also best to choose low-salt or unsalted nuts to reduce sodium intake.

Here is a list of nutrient-dense nuts to work into your daily diet:

- Almonds
- Brazil nuts
- Cashews
- Hazelnuts
- Macadamia nuts
- Peanuts – botanically a legume but culinary considered a nut
- Pecans
- Pine nuts
- Pistachio nuts
- Walnuts

Legumes for Brain Longevity

Legumes, also known as pulses, include all types of beans, peas, lentils, and chickpeas and are found in a variety of forms – dried, canned, cooked and frozen.

Many cultures throughout the world use legumes as an important part of their diet and for those that do, longevity is a major health benefit. For example, people in Japan enjoy a longer lifespan because of soybean-derived foods such as tofu, natto and miso, as do people in the Mediterranean where lentils, chickpeas, and white beans are a mainstay.[32]

Legumes are a nutrient rich, low-fat source of protein, fiber, B vitamins, minerals such as iron, zinc, calcium, and magnesium, as well as many phytonutrients. Economical, versatile, and easy to prepare, legumes have been a main source of protein for anyone following a vegan diet but anyone vegan or not, can enjoy the nutritional package legumes have to offer.

As far as the benefit to brain health, legumes have been shown to play a role in slowing cognitive decline. A study of more than 2,000 Swedish older adults aged 60 and up showed that those who regularly consumed beans had better cognition which was believed to be partly from beans neuroprotection.[33]

Besides brain benefits, legumes are a low-glycemic, slow-digesting carbohydrate food ideal for controlling blood glucose for those with diabetes. Additionally, high fiber, high potassium, and zero cholesterol content makes legumes heart healthy.

Legumes can be easily added into many dishes to boost fiber, protein, and phytonutrient content. Here are some ideas to get you started:

- Anytime you have a salad, add beans to provide texture, taste and dimension

- Spread sandwiches with hummus made from chickpeas in place of mayonnaise

- Add beans, lentils, or split peas to soups such as minestrone or tomato

- Add black beans to scrambled eggs

- Add beans, split peas or lentils to whole dishes such as quinoa or brown rice pilaf

- Cooked lentils can be added to pancake batter or oatmeal for a more crunchy taste and texture

Most of us fall short on eating a sufficient amount of legumes in our diet. Make it a habit to begin including more legumes by consuming at least four ½ cup servings each week. Choose from among these nutrient-rich legumes:

- Beans — black, butter, cannellini, chickpeas, fava, great northern, kidney, lima, navy, pinto, red, and white
- Black-eyed peas
- Edamame (soybeans)
- Lentils
- Split peas
- Tofu

Healthy Fats for Brain Health –
Fish, Oils, Poultry, Red Meat

Healthy fats have been found to have a significant positive impact on keeping your brain sharp and functioning at its best.[34] The key of course is "healthy" fats. This section will focus on specific foods which contain healthier monounsaturated and polyunsaturated fats.

FISH – A good catch for brain health is fatty fish. Why? Because fatty fish are rich in the all-important omega-3 fatty acid called *docosahexaenoic acid* or DHA which has been shown to help improve memory in adults and is critical for the brain and eye development in babies. Deep-water fish such as salmon are brimming with essential omega-3 fatty acids necessary for brain functioning. Omega-3's also contain anti-inflammatory substances that protect the brain and keep it mentally sharp.

These same omega-3 fatty acids found in fatty fish also are key to a healthy cardiovascular system that supplies blood and nutrients to the brain. In fact, one study found eating one serving of fatty fish a week is associated with a 7% lower risk of Alzheimer's disease compared to not eating fish.[35]

Since numerous studies have demonstrated the beneficial effects of fatty fish for heart health, the American Heart Association recommends eating two 3 to 5-ounce servings of fatty fish each week.

The best fatty fish to choose from for improving brain and your heart health include:

- Anchovies
- Halibut
- Herring
- Mackerel
- Salmon
- Sardines
- Trout
- Tuna

OILS – An important source of our healthy fats come from vegetable oils. Vegetables oils are predominantly composed of monounsaturated and polyunsaturated fats and an excellent source of vitamin E and plant-based omega-3 fatty acids, all important for protecting brain health.

Scientific studies have shown how vitamin E and omega-3 fatty acids are associated with promoting good brain health and lowering the risk of dementia.

However, one oil in particular rises to the top – olive oil. The MIND diet highly recommends the use of olive oil as part of a brain-healthy diet.

When shopping for olive oil, choose "extra-virgin." Extra virgin olive oil has an excellent fat profile in that it contains high levels of *oleic acid*, about 75% compared to 60% found in canola and corn oils. Oleic acid is a monounsaturated fat helping reduce overall blood cholesterol levels by lowering unhealthy LDL cholesterol. Another characteristic of extra virgin olive oil setting it apart from other oils is its extremely high level of polyphenols. These compounds act as antioxidants protecting cells against unwanted inflammation and disease. Extra virgin olive oil contains more polyphenols than other olive oils. This same oil also boasts high levels of the antioxidant vitamin E that protects cells from damaging free radicals.

According to the California Olive Oil council, "extra virgin" is the highest grade an oil can receive. Olive oil is considered "extra virgin" when it has been produced by a simple pressing of the olives.

Extra virgin olive oil comes from the unprocessed fruit of olive trees. When processed, the fruit is simply crushed to extract the oil content at a temperature no higher than 86 degrees Fahrenheit.

This helps preserve the olive's nutritional benefits. This minimal processing essentially means olive oil is a fruit juice. Oils such as corn, canola, soybean, and other vegetable oils have to go through several steps from being chemically-extracted, refined, bleached and deodorized.

Other grades of olive oil simply labeled as "olive oil" and not labeled as "extra virgin olive oil," are usually produced using chemicals and extreme heat during the extraction process which is what makes extra virgin olive oil special. It has not gone through the refining process which destroys polyphenols through oxidation. The label of "extra virgin" also indicates that the oil is free flavor or odor defects.

Unfortunately, you may be standing in the grocery store ready to buy an olive oil stating "extra virgin," when in fact, it may be adulterated with refined oil or made with low-standard production practices. Since the industry isn't regulated, a bottle of olive oil claiming it has been imported from Italy, does not guarantee a high-quality olive oil.

The best way to know you are buying authentic extra virgin olive oil with the healthiest nutritional value is to look for certification seals by national and state olive oil associations such as the California Olive Oil Council (COOC) or the Italian Agricultural Confederation (CIA).

Other oils to consider that are nutrient dense include the following:

- Canola (rapeseed)
- Corn
- Cottonseed
- Grapeseed
- Olive
- Peanut
- Safflower
- Sesame
- Soybean
- Sunflower
- Walnut

POULTRY – Scientific evidence of poultry's contribution to improving cognitive functioning is minimal, but the MIND diet does recommend eating poultry twice a week. Poultry is a healthy source of protein and an excellent source of B vitamins such as vitamin B12, an essential nutrient that has been shown to play a part in brain health.

Like all animal sources of protein, poultry is considered a high-quality protein meaning that it contains all nine of the essential amino acids. The most commonly consumed poultry are chicken and turkey. When choosing poultry, skinless meat from the breast will be leaner than dark meat from the thighs. If buying ground chicken or turkey, choose 90 to 95 percent lean options.

Many groceries now offer rotisserie chicken and sometimes turkey, a convenient, ready-to-go food. However, look for no-salt-added options and avoid ones that state "savory" or "juicy" which are often code words for "pumped with added sodium." Remove the skin and any visible fat.

The MIND diet and the American Heart Association recommend poultry without the skin, baked or grilled, twice a week.

RED MEAT – Say "red meat" and most people will assume you are talking about beef. But beef is not the only meat considered "red." Red meat refers to all types of mammalian muscle meat which includes not only beef but also veal, bison, pork, lamb, and goat. These meats are called "red" because they contain more myoglobin than "white" meats of poultry or fish. Myoglobin is a protein in meat which holds the oxygen in the muscle.

People often associate all red meat with being a less healthy form of protein. But the idea that all red meat is less healthful than white meat is not true.

Researchers at Purdue University have found a Mediterranean-style diet can improve the wellness of your heart without cutting out red meat altogether.[36] This study focused on whether eating red meat resulted in increasing the risk for cardiovascular disease. Results showed if the red meat is lean and unprocessed, it had a neutral effect neither increasing or lowering heart disease. Therefore, for those who enjoy eating red meat, as long as it's lean red meat, it can be part of a healthy diet.

So, how does eating red meat benefit your brain? There is little scientific research showing red meat's effect on brain health. However, there are several studies that do show lean red meat's positive effect on heart health. And what's good for the heart, is good for the brain.

Lean red meats sources are a naturally nutrient-rich source of many nutrients including high-quality protein, iron, zinc, and many B-vitamins. It is one of the best sources to help you meet your nutritional needs.

Take beef for example. A 2012 study found that people who consumed 4 to 5.5 ounces of lean beef daily as part of the heart-healthy Beef in an Optimal Lean Diet (BOLD), had a 10 percent decline in LDL or "bad" cholesterol as well as a reduction in total cholesterol.[37] These results are similar to what has been observed for the DASH diet.

The fatty acids in a serving of beef are heart-healthy monounsaturated fatty acids, the same type found in olive oil. In addition, nearly one-third of the saturated fat in lean beef is stearic acid, a fatty acid shown to have neutral effects on cholesterol levels.

The key factor in eating red meat such as beef is to know how "lean beef" is defined. The United States Department of Agricultural defines lean beef as a 3 ounce serving of cooked beef with less than 10 grams of total, fat, 4.5 grams or less of saturated fat, and less than 95 milligrams of cholesterol.

Another important takeaway about red meat is to limit the frequency of consuming it to no more than two servings a week.

When at the grocery store, you need to know how to identify "lean" red meat. Below are examples of what to look for, what the healthiest cooking methods are, and what a proper portion should be:

- Look for cuts with the words, "round" or "loin" in the name.

  For beef - choose lean cuts such as eye of round roast or steak, sirloin tip side steak, top round roast or steak, or top sirloin steak.

  For bison – sirloin, rib eye, and top round all have 2 grams of fat per serving.

  For veal – leg, sirloin, and loin all have 3 grams or less fat per serving.

  For pork – tenderloin has 2 grams of fat per serving and sirloin has 4 grams of fat per serving.

  For lamb – lamb shank, loin, and shoulder have 6 grams of fat or less per serving.

- For ground beef, choose 96 percent extra lean (4 percent of fat).

- Trim off any excess fat before cooking.

- Broil, bake, or grill red meat; avoid frying.

- Enjoy small portions. An appropriate portion size for lean red meat is about 3-4 ounces or the size of a smart phone or the size and thickness of the palm of your hand.

Brain-Draining Foods

Now that we've covered foods promoting brain health, you'll need to know what foods may harm the health of your brain. Of course, there will be times when these not-so-healthy foods will part served at a holiday, birthday celebration, wedding, funeral, or any other sort of occasion. To completely eliminate these foods is unrealistic. The occasional treat here and there can be enjoyed as long as it doesn't become an everyday indulge fest overtaking the brain healthy foods completely.

As we go through the list of foods to avoid, many of them are loaded with excess sodium, unhealthy saturated and or trans fats or too much sugar. These food substances are known for increasing inflammation, raising blood lipids to unhealthy levels, and increasing your risk of developing heart disease, obesity, diabetes, hypertension, and stroke. When you have the option to choose a food promoting your cognitive health or one that does not, do the smart thing by eating what enhances your brain.

Unhealthy Fats

The type of fat you use is important. Whatever you cook with, use as a spread, or dip bread into, fats make a difference. Fat is a necessary component of your diet as it performs many functions in your body but it's all about feeding your body the best fat it requires for optimal health.

One of the most talked about types of fat in recent years is coconut oil. If you read the headlines, you'd believe coconut oil is a miracle food and the next best thing to olive oil. Touted as "the oil that can do it all," coconut oil fanatics have made claims that it can lower your risk of heart disease, cancer, and even prevent Alzheimer's disease. But what is remarkable is that there is very little evidence to support these claims.

As far as coconut oil as brain fuel, proponents say that it has a high percentage of medium-chain triglycerides (MCTs), a type of fat metabolized differently than long-chain triglycerides (LCT) a type of fat found in the majority of liquid oils. The claim is that MCTs can treat Alzheimer's and restore some brain function. Studies that have reviewed this claim have found no support from any large, peer-reviewed clinical trials saying that coconut oil is effective for treating Alzheimer's disease.[38]

What about butter and stick margarine? The MIND diet discourages the use of these products to no more than a tablespoon per day. Fats that are solid at room temperature such as butter and stick margarine contain too much saturated fat.

Here is a listing of fats to reduce your intake of to a minimum:

- Beef tallow
- Butter
- Coconut oil
- Lard
- Palm oil
- Shortening
- Stick margarine

Whole-Fat Cheese

It's no surprise that the biggest contributor of saturated fat in the American diet is cheese. We love to pile it on pizza, serve it as a dip with tortilla chips, and top a burger with several slices. We love our cheese. Unfortunately, it's loaded with saturated fat. Just a one ounce serving of American cheese has more saturated fat (5.1 grams) than a serving of lean roast beef (3.4 grams). In 2016, the annual per capita consumption of cheese in the United States was 38.5 pounds.

Very few of us do not like cheese – cheddar and mozzarella are our favorites. But for the sake and health of your brain, you have to think of cheese as an accent to a meal or an occasional treat. Instead of loading up your pizza with extra cheese, if making your own, be creative and opt for extra virgin olive oil while piling on the veggies.

Even I like cheese and nothing says "comfort" more than a grilled cheddar cheese sandwich, especially on cold, winter days. But, on the infrequent occasions I do have one, I make sure to add on a sliced tomato and have a side spinach salad loaded with other vegetables.

The rule of thumb for how much cheese we can enjoy without going overboard is to limit whole-fat cheese consumption to 2 ounces each week. To eyeball what a portion of a 2 ounce serving of hard cheese looks like, this is equivalent to the size of a domino; a 1 ounce serving of hard cheese is about the size of your thumb or 2 tablespoons of crumbled cheese such as feta.

Below is a table showing you the amount of saturated and total fat in various cheeses. Notice that hard cheese such as Cheddar, Colby, and Swiss, are highest in saturated fat.

Cheese (each 1 ounce)	Saturated fat (grams)	Total fat (grams)
Cheddar	5.3	9.4
Colby	5.7	9.1
Swiss	5.2	8.8
American	5.1	8.6
Goat	5.8	8.5
Blue	5.3	8.1
Gouda	5.0	7.8
Mozzarella	3.7	6.3
Feta	4.2	6.0

Source: United States Department of Agriculture, National Agriculture Library

To significantly reduce total and saturated fat content in cheese, consider using low-fat cheeses. Part-skim mozzarella cheese will reduce saturated fat by 20 percent while part-skim ricotta cheese will reduce saturated fat by 40 percent. Or replace ricotta cheese with low-fat cottage cheese (which has only 0.7 grams of saturated fat per ½ cup) for an even better reduction of unhealthy fat.

Pastries, Sweets and Sugary Beverages

Americans love their sweets. So much so that it's been implicated as a major villain leading to increases in weight gain and obesity, type 2 diabetes, and heart disease.

The average American consumes 22 teaspoons of added sugar each day coming from pastries, sweets, and sugary beverages. A study called the National Health and Nutrition Examination Survey (NHANES) III from 1988 to 2006, compared participants who consumed less than 10 percent of their calories from added sugar to those who consumed 25 percent or more, those who ate 25 percent of more of their calories from added sugar had nearly three times the risk of death from cardiovascular diseases over 15 years.[39] In fact, the Healthy People 2020 objectives have recommended that Americans should keep their intake of added sugars to less than 10 percent of their total daily calories as part of a healthy diet.[40] For example, in a 2,000 daily calorie diet no more than 200 calories should come from added sugars.

Even though there is no direct scientific evidence that eliminating sugary foods and beverages will protect you from developing dementia or Alzheimer's, there are still many of reasons why you should limit these foods.

One reason is many of these foods are referred to as "empty calorie" foods - Empty calorie foods are foods where the majority of calories are from unhealthy ingredients – solid fats like shortening or butter, added sugar that only add calories to a food but with few or no nutrients.

For instance, drinking a can of soda is an empty calorie food. It contains lots of sugar, water, and that's it. No vitamins, minerals, fiber, or protein. If your main source of calories is coming from overly sugary foods and beverages, you're getting little nutritional bang for your buck.

Because these empty calorie foods offer too many calories, sugar and oftentimes too much fat, you will not be helping feed your brain the antioxidants, phytochemicals, and other substances that support cognitive functioning. These same foods can also lead to blood sugar spikes that lead to inflammation that damages arteries of the heart.

I'm sure many of you already know but the foods listed below are prime examples of what is considered pastries, sweets, and sugary beverages:

- Brownies
- Cake
- Candy
- Cookies
- Croissants
- Cupcakes
- Doughnuts
- Ice cream
- Lemonade
- Pastries
- Sugar-sweetened beverages such as soda, sports drinks, any juice that is not 100 percent fruit juice

There are certainly many more foods that could be added to this list but this gives you the idea of which foods you should curb your intake. The recommendation is to have no more than five servings a week of any of these foods – the less, the better.

Fried Foods and Fast Foods

Last on the list of brain-draining foods but certainly not least, are fried foods and fast foods. It should be no surprise these foods are under the headline of foods harmful to brain health.

Anyone who eats a steady diet of burgers, French fries, fried chicken, fried fish, hush puppies, mozzarella sticks or any other food that can be deep fried (which is almost anything), is doing their body few favors.

Deep frying is a common cooking method used around the world. Often used by restaurants and fast food chains, deep frying is a quick and inexpensive way to prepare foods, at the sake of your health.

What makes fried foods and fast foods detrimental to your health? Compared to other cooking methods, frying adds a lot of calories.

Typically fried foods are coated in batter or flour prior to being cooked. When foods are fried in oil, they lose water and absorb fat, which further increases their calorie and fat content, much more so when compared to other foods.[41] This can significantly increase one's risk for developing heart disease, type 2 diabetes, stroke, and obesity.

Those of you relying on fast food to get you through each week, beware. Too many trips through the drive-thru put you at risk of missing out on essential micronutrients such as vitamin A and C, carotenoids, magnesium, and calcium – some of which are necessary for good brain health.

Fast food restaurants are well aware that the American public is showing more interest in what kind of nutritional bang for their buck they're getting. Because of this, attempts have been made by these restaurants to offer the public more healthy options such as salads, fruit and grilled items like chicken. However, the MIND diet still recommends limiting fried fast food to less than one serving a week or to limit eating at these establishments no more than twice a month.

The best bet when eating at a fast food restaurant is to go for the healthiest options on the menu. Choose a salad with toppings and dressing on the side, grilled chicken or grilled fish on whole wheat bread, or a healthier side such as baby carrots or apple slices instead of French fries. Your body and your brain will thank you for feeding it food that will nourish it best.

CHAPTER SIX

MEAL PLANNING TO MAXIMIZE BRAIN HEALTH

"The signs of my husband's early-onset Alzheimer's were everywhere. In the beginning, I noticed little changes such as asking me the same questions over and over. Then, bigger, more dangerous changes starting happening – driving down the wrong side of the road or forgetting to turn off the stove. One day I went to a neighbor's house for about 10 minutes. When I returned home, the door was locked and he was nowhere in sight. I didn't have my house key so I knocked on the front door repeatedly, called my home phone with my cell phone, honked on the car horn but he wouldn't respond. Finally, he came to the door, puzzled as to where I had been. I had told him where I was going but he simply said, 'No, you were in the bathtub a few minutes ago.' It was when his employer required him to visit his doctor and then admitted to the hospital for a 10-day observational stay, that he was given the diagnosis of Alzheimer's."

-Brenda
Wife and caretaker of her husband, Loren, who was
diagnosed with Alzheimer's disease at the age of 57

Now you're ready to put all this information into practice. You want the best for your brain. It all begins with smart eating by meal planning. This means making most, if not every bite count. When you implement what you've learned so far, you'll start choosing foods that nourish brain health helping you get the best it deserves.

Following a brain-healthy diet is not hard to do. The previous chapters have laid the groundwork of what foods are the most healthy and most harmful to your brain and why. All you need to do is decide what foods go on your plate, and when you have chosen well, the nutrients essential for preserving cognitive function, will do their part. The good thing about this way of eating is that you do not need to worry about counting calories or grams of specific nutrients (unless you have a disease such as diabetes).

The Essentials of Meal Planning

One of the best tools everyone single one of us can do to enhance our overall health is to plan our meals. Anyone who flies by the seat of their pants with no idea of what to have for dinner whenever 5 pm rolls around, likely will resort to fast food as the answer. Convenient, yes, but night after night of picking up dinner at a drive-thru window is no friend to your health, particularly your brain health.

Meal planning may sound old-fashioned but it has become more in-fashion as an excellent means of eating a balanced diet and for meeting your nutritional needs. And what every seasoned meal planner will tell you, meal planning also saves you time and money.

When you take some time to plan meals for the week, you already know what your meals will look like and what foods you need to buy. A good spin-off of meal planning is taking your grocery list with you when buying food which automatically reduces impulse purchases.

Meal Planning Basics

This is where the fun begins and yes, meal planning can be fun and enjoyable. Whether you are a Martha Stewart or Julia Child in the kitchen or more of a beginner, planning meals can be as simple or elaborate as you want. Here's how to start:

- Ask your family to suggest meal ideas.
- For inspiration, flip through cookbooks or check out recipe websites. There are even sample menus and menu-planning apps online.

- Home cooking doesn't have to be elaborate. Focus on a handful of recipes that you can rotate through for most of your meals.

- Cooking from scratch can get healthy meals on the table but so can taking shortcuts. For instance, pair home-cooked foods with healthy store-bought staples to save on time without compromising on nutrition. Think pasta with marinara sauce in a jar, soup with canned beans, or pre-chopped spinach and rotisserie chicken with prewashed greens.

- Most people who practice meal planning only plan their main meal each day. If dinner is the main meal for your family, then plan 5-7 dinner meals for the week. Or, if you have more time, you can plan breakfast, lunch and dinner for as many days a week as you want.

- Plan a week of meals at a time. Start with the entrée or main dish and include side dishes to go along with it.

- Once your menu ideas are filled in, create a shopping list of the ingredients you'll need.

- Coordinate your meal planning with other activities and meetings you have throughout each week. Check your calendar to decide which nights you will only have time to reheat leftovers.

- To keep meal planning entertaining and rewarding, think seasonal. What fresh produce is available at certain times of the year? Is it salad weather or soup season?

- Mix things up by planning meatless meals or trying out new recipes and old favorites.

- Keep a visual in your mind of what each meal will look like on your plate. Are there sufficient colors and textures or is everything you planned bland and uninteresting ?

- Planning meals around themes helps make the planning process flow. For example, maybe Monday nights are always pasta night and Thursday nights are always fish night. Or, one night can be designated "cook's choice." Use that night to clean out your refrigerator by making a stir-fry, omelets, or chef salad.

• The nice thing about meal planning is that you can recycle your plans.

• Most of all learn to be flexible. Even your best thought out plans can get disrupted as no meal plan is set in stone.

One of the best ways to keep your meal planning organized is to download or create a meal plan template. Here is one example of a brain-healthy foods menu for one week could look like for you and your family:

	BREAKFAST	LUNCH	DINNER	SNACKS
MONDAY	Greek yogurt with berries and walnuts, cubed cantaloupe	Veggie Split Pea Soup (pg 96), leafy green salad	Mediterranean salmon (pg 84), brown rice with beans, baked apple with cherries and almonds	Tangerine slices and popcorn
TUESDAY	Whole grain cereal with milk, fruit	Vegetable pasta primavera (pg 88), blackberries or strawberries	Walnut-crusted chicken (pg 81), baked sweet potato, broccoli	Unsalted almonds, fresh veggies with hummus
WEDNESDAY	Grab-n-go mini breakfast casseroles (pg 79) with orange slices	Tuna or salmon edamame salad with pita bread	Beef top sirloin and fruit kabobs (pg 83), grilled corn	Blueberries or blackberries with walnuts and cashew sweet cream (pg 107)
THURSDAY	Berry banana smoothie with whole grain toast	Mixed leafy greens, pecans, pumpkin seeds, dried cranberries	Baked halibut, wheat berry salad, asparagus	Sliced apples with cubed cheese
FRIDAY	Scrambled eggs, oatmeal with berries	Turkey sandwich, cut raw veggies like carrots and zucchini, strawberries	Roasted chicken, broccoli and barley pilaf, sautéed leafy greens	Bean dip with whole grain crackers

How to Eyeball the Perfect Portion Size of Food

It's one thing to know how to meal plan but it's also wise to know what a proper portion size of food should look like. Portion distortion, mainly due to huge restaurant portion sizes distorting our view of what a normal amount of food should be, has been a problem for decades.

Below is a table showing types of food and how to use visuals keeping your portions sizes reasonable to enhance your health:

Food	Serving Size
Vegetables	1 cup fresh leafy greens, ½ cup cooked leafy greens, ½ cup other vegetables
Fruit	½ cup fresh berries, 1 small piece of fruit, ¼ cup dried fruit
Whole grains	½ cup cooked
Nuts	¼ cup or 1 ounce
Beans	½ cup cooked
Fish, Poultry, Red Meat	3 ounces
Olive oil	1 tablespoon
Cheese	1 ounce
Milk, Yogurt	1 cup

When it comes to estimating portions, visual cues help. When filling your plate, picture these items to remind you of proper serving sizes:

- **Vegetables (raw leafy vegetables, 2 cups; cooked leafy vegetables or other vegetables, ½ cup):**
  For one cup – A tennis ball
  For ½ cup – Half of a tennis ball

- **Fruit (dried fruit, ¼ cup, fresh or frozen, ½ cup):**
  For ¼ cup – A ping pong ball or a large egg
  For ½ cup – Half of a tennis ball

- **Grains (pasta, rice, cereal, cooked grains, ½ cup):**
  Half of a tennis ball

- **Nuts – (¼ cup):**
  Shot glass
  Medium egg

- **Beans – (½ cup):**
  Half of a tennis ball

- **Protein (meat, fish, poultry, 3 ounces):**
  Smartphone
  Palm of your hand (no fingers)
  Deck of cards

- **All oils – (1 tablespoon):**
  The size of one thumb where it bends to the tip

- **Cheese – (1 ounce):**
  A pair of dice

- **Milk, yogurt – (1 cup):**
  A tennis ball

Stocking a Brain-Healthy Kitchen

To feed your brain what it needs for improved cognitive functioning, brain-enhancing foods need to be on hand in your kitchen. What you buy at the grocery store, bring home, and then store in your pantry, refrigerator and freezer, will be the base of what you have to work with so choose wisely. When nourishing, healthy foods are already on hand, it takes out much of the guesswork and uncertainty of what to have for meals. Here is a good start of foods to have available:

In Your Cupboards and Pantry

Vegetables - Canned vegetables such as green beans, corn, and tomatoes (whole, diced, crushed, pureed, or made into a paste)

Fruit – Canned fruit (unsweetened or packed with water or own juice) such as peaches, pears, apricots, and applesauce

Beans – Canned or dried beans – such as black, butter, cannellini, chickpeas, fava, great northern, kidney, lima, navy, pinto, red, and white; also soybeans, peas, and lentils

Nuts – Almonds, Brazil nuts, cashews, hazelnuts, macadamia nuts, peanuts, pecans, pine nuts, pistachios, and walnuts

Seeds – Chia, flaxseed, pumpkin, sesame, and sunflower seeds

Fish – Canned tuna, salmon, anchovy, sardines, and herring

Oils – Extra-virgin olive oil, canola, corn, cottonseed, grapeseed, peanut, safflower, sesame, soybean, sunflower, and walnut.

Whole grains – Amaranth, barley, buckwheat, brown and wild rice, bulgur, corn, farro, freekeh, kamut berries, kaniwa, millet, oats, popcorn, quinoa, rye, sorghum, spelt, teff, triticale, and wheat berries.

In Your Freezer

Vegetables – Broccoli, carrots, cauliflower, corn, edamame, green beans, kale, peas, and spinach

Fruit – Blueberries, raspberries, mangoes, strawberries (unsweetened), and tart cherries

Nuts – Nuts can go rancid quickly due to their high oil content. It's recommended to store nuts in the freezer if you don't plan on using them right away. To freeze peanuts, walnuts, almonds, pecans, cashews, macadamia nuts, and hazelnuts, wrap well in plastic, then place in a resealable freezer bag.

Meat – Have on hand lean red meat, poultry without the skin and fish high in omega-3 fatty acids

All fish, poultry and red meat not being used right away should be stored in the freezer

In Your Refrigerator

Vegetables – Artichokes, asparagus, beets, green beans, bell peppers, Brussel sprouts, broccoli, cabbage, carrots, cauliflower, celery, cut vegetables, herbs, mushrooms, peas, radishes, sprouts, summer squashes, sweet corn, and all leafy greens.

Certain vegetables are best kept out of the refrigerator including onions, potatoes, garlic, and tomatoes. Refrigeration can damage the quality of their taste of these vegetables when cooked due to the changes that occur in the composition of the carbohydrate they contain.

As long as these vegetables are whole and freshly harvested or picked up at the grocery store, they shouldn't go into the refrigerator as they may also need more time to ripen. However, once these particular vegetables have been cut, then store in the refrigerator for food safety.

To properly store onions and garlic, place in separate mesh bags, a wire basket or a crate allowing air circulation, in a cool, dry location such as a basement (32 to 40 degrees Fahreneheit). Potatoes are best kept in a well-ventilated container and stored in a dry location away from sunlight at temperatures between 45 and 55 degrees Fahrenheit. Ripe tomatoes should be kept at room temperature away from sunlight.

Fruit – All berries, apples, apricots, figs, grapes, and any cut fruit.

CHAPTER SEVEN

LEADING A BRAIN-HEALTHY LIFESTYLE

"It was my Dad who first noticed the gradual loss of my Mom's memory. The signs and symptoms she exhibited were indicative of the features of Alzheimer's disease. After her diagnosis, Dad started to read several books about Mom's condition which he shared with her. I had strong doubts that even if Mom had read any of the books that she wouldn't be able to fully comprehend how the information related to her. Within time, Mom was unable to complete full sentences or carry on a conversation. Since my family had been filling in the gaps of when she had memory loss, interactions with Mom felt fairly normal allowing me to convince myself she wasn't aware of her decline. One day when we were alone, Mom looked at me and said, 'I wonder what happens when they can't talk anymore?' I realized at that point she was recalling something she had heard or read about her disease and when she said 'they' she really meant 'me.' She knew."

-Toni
Daughter of Velma, who was diagnosed
with Alzheimer's disease at the age of 76.

A brain-healthy diet is just one piece of the puzzle for reducing, delaying and preferably avoiding Alzheimer's disease and other forms of dementia. Learning and then making changes to your dietary choices is an important first step in keeping your brain sharp. Besides dietary changes, other valuable lifestyle modifications also help round out what you can do to preserve and protect your brain from dementia.

Fortunately, research keeps paving the way providing clues to age-proofing your brain. David A. Bennett, MD, director of the Rush Alzheimer's Disease Center in Chicago - along with about 100 scientists - has been searching for ways to treat and prevent a range of common neurodegenerative disorders.

For almost 25 years Bennett has led two longitudinal investigations – the Religious Orders Study and the Rush Memory and Aging Project – enrolling more than 3,200 dementia-free adults from across the United States ranging in age from mid-50s to their 100s.[42,43] Their aim was to pinpoint why some people stay sharp into old age while others lose their mental faculties as early as their 50's. All of the volunteers agreed to donate their brains after death for the scientists to research.

Bennett and his team discovered that it was rare for just about anyone to grow old with a completely healthy brain. Almost every single brain they examined exhibited at least some form of the neuron-killing tangles associated with Alzheimer's disease.

Not all of those with these tangles, however, further advanced to show signs of the disease. This begs the question of why some people develop symptoms of Alzheimer's while others do not?

Your brain is the most adaptable of all organs. It can fight back drawing on its cognitive reserves to stop Alzheimer's from advancing further. This is where each and every one of us can help this process along in our day-to-day living. Like me, maybe you didn't win the genetic lottery of having few if any family members escaping dementia. You may believe that only the inevitable will happen just like it did for your relatives.

This is where tangible and useful information from researchers across the world working diligently to unlock the key to preventing Alzheimer's and dementia is priceless.

A main takeaway from the two longitudinal studies were 10 key lifestyle factors that do shape our brain's health into old age, making it difficult for Alzheimer's and other forms of dementia to make an appearance.

These 10 factors have been identified as playing a vital role in building a better brain by certain lifestyle choices and activities we engage in.

Here are the ten lifestyle factors to consider for protecting brain health:

1. Keep learning throughout life – From the day we are born to the day we die, there is always something new we can learn. Lifelong learning and education can secure brain health as you age. Even though you may believe you already know everything, there is always something new to discover. Learning a second language, taking music or art lessons, or taking up an activity such as gardening can help avoid emotional and mental neglect.

2. Engage in regular cognitive and physical activity – To maintain brain health means to engage your brain with cognitively stimulating activities. This may sound rather intimidating but it boils down to any opportunities that keep your mind active as you age. These activities run the gamut from mental challenges such as playing chess or checkers, to rearranging furniture. In general, all adults, no matter what age, should be encouraged to engage their mind by trying new and challenging activities that promote their cognitive and overall health.[44]

Physical activity is another vital factor in keeping your mind healthy. Not only is it necessary to keep yourself physically fit but your brain benefits from the workout, too.

Researchers from the University of Kansas Alzheimer's Disease Center conducted a study that found people who walked briskly for 20 to 25 minutes several times a week – achievable for most of us – showed improvements in their thinking skills, especially in regards to attention and creating visual maps of spaces in their heads. These two cognitive abilities are often known to decline as you age.[45]

Other research has found regular aerobic exercise, the kind that gets your blood pumping, appears to boost the size of the hippocampus, the brain area involved in verbal memory and learning.[46] Investing in "sweat equity" can also pay off in better brain health by reducing insulin resistance, inflammation, and stimulation of growth factors that affect the health of brain cells. In addition, moving your body more improves mood and sleep while reducing stress and anxiety, factors which frequently contribute to cognitive decline.

How much exercise is required to improve memory? It is recommended to achieve moderate physical activity of at least 30 minutes on most days of the week. This can include taking a brisk walk, swimming, playing tennis or putting on music and dancing. One study found dancing to be a dynamic deterrent for decreasing dementia.[47] It showed that older people who routinely danced had an increased size in the hippocampus region of the brain, which plays a key role in memory and learning, as well as keeping one's balance. Even active household chores can count as well such as raking leaves, push mowing a lawn, or intense floor mopping.

3. Strengthen and maintain social ties – Strong friendships make for a better brain. Our brains are wired to connect with others. As humans, we have a basic need to belong to a group and form bonds with one another. Whether it's being in a loving relationship, socializing with classmates, at school, participating in civic or religious groups, these connections with others have an impressive impact on our brain health. Studies have found that maintaining strong social networks appears to slow down cognitive decline.[48] You don't have to be the life of the party, but do be present and engage with those around you.

4. Get out and explore new things – The word "explore" can have different meanings for different people. For some it may literally mean stuffing a backpack with essentials and spending weeks traveling by foot in a foreign country. For others, it could be as simple as exploring a nature trail just down the road they may have not traveled yet. The main idea is to challenge your brain. Expand your mind by doing something new that tests your mental skills. Take a cooking class, learn ballroom dancing, join a book club, become a museum docent, or teach others a new skill. Anything that stimulates brain activity is beneficial.

Even using everyday tasks to forge new brain cell connections are helpful. As an example, brush your teeth with the hand you normally don't use. Take a different route to work or the grocery store. If the only music you listen to is rock and roll, turn the dial to classical music for ten minutes a day. Do 60 seconds of jumping jacks (or other physical activities). Sit in a different chair in your house. Make it a habit of doing one new thing each day.

5. Relax and be happy – The song, *"Don't Worry, Be Happy,"* has a memorable line - "Listen to what I say, in your life expect some trouble, but when you worry, you make it double." Stress is a given. None of us will get through life without it. What matters is how you handle and manage it. If you let stress consume your mental energy, this can lead to anxiety and depression, both bad for brain health. But when you learn and use relaxation strategies, it makes a big difference in your mind and mood. Each day, spend 10 minutes sitting or lying down relaxed with your eyes closed, focusing on your breathing and relaxing your body. Regular meditation helps keep your brain healthier and happier.

Happiness can mean different things to different people, but a large part of it is staying positive and being resilient. When you can bounce back from difficult situations, it often predicts how satisfied you are in life. Factors that help you achieve this are surrounding yourself with positivity. From encouraging co-workers, family and friends, to finding something humorous every day to laugh about, each can boost self-esteem while giving your brain a break from stress, worry, and anxiety.

6. Avoid people who are downers – No one likes or prefers to spend time with those who make us feel diminished, sad, scared, worried, angry, or depressed, especially if they are family members. Each of us only has one life to live. Make the most of your precious time by filling your life with meaningful and healthy relationships.

7. Be conscientious and diligent – "Conscientious" is a big word, but it is considered one of the most desirable personality traits one can have. Being a conscientious person means being mindful of those around you from friends and family to colleagues and even strangers. If you are someone who likes to make a good first impression when introduced to new people, you likely have this trait. You also likely are well-organized and tidy, reliable, driven by personal goals and plan well into the future.

The trait of being diligent goes hand-in-hand with being a conscientious person. If you are diligent, you share many of the qualities of being conscientious but with a caring streak that bubbles over into your work and other activities you do.

So, how does this help brain health? Conscientious, and diligent people, who are also punctual, studious, and ethical, have been found to have greater strength of the wiring connections between brain regions.

This payoff results in the fact that conscientiousness is good for your health in terms of longevity and in addition to being beneficial for your brain.[49]

8. Spend time engaged in activities that are meaningful and goal-oriented – Do you know what your purpose in life is? It's a question all of us should contemplate. Researchers at the Rush Alzheimer's Disease Center have studied this very question suggesting that having a strong purpose in life might be neuroprotective or brain-preserving. Their studies have found that older adults who felt useless or with little purpose in life were more likely to develop Alzheimer's disease than those with a strong sense of purpose in life.[50]

Participation in meaningful work or activities oriented towards achieving a specific goal can be very rewarding. The sense of belonging, accomplishment, and making life better for others, is bound to make you feel purposeful sparking motivation, ambition, and perseverance.

Maintaining positivity about aging is crucial for not becoming negative about life. The power of positive thinking and optimism is so pivotal that people, who see the glass as half full as opposed to half empty are significantly less likely to develop dementia than pessimistic people.[51]

Each of us must carve out our purpose in life. Finding your niche, what is it that inspires passion in you, may be one factor that drives dementia away.

9. Be heart-healthy – What's good for the heart is good for the brain. What you should be doing for heart health – exercising and eating a healthy diet – are also key factors in helping reduce your risk of Alzheimer's disease and other forms of dementia.

Since your brain is one of the most active organs in your body, it makes sense to pay attention to your heart health. Each day, your heart pumps about 20% of your blood to your brain, where oxygen and food are used. Any condition that damages the blood vessels in your brain or keeps your heart from pumping efficiently can deprive your brain from getting the nutrients it needs and stop new brain cells from forming. Obesity, high cholesterol, and high blood pressure have all been linked to a higher risk of Alzheimer's disease. Eating a healthy diet and regular physical exercise will keep your brain healthier as you age, as well as reduce your risk for heart attack, stroke, and diabetes.

10. Eat a MIND diet, with fresh fruit, vegetables, and fish – One of the most consistent messages and recommendations for maintaining brain health is to adopt a healthy diet. The specifics of "brain protective" diets vary but tend to have certain elements in common – consume a diet higher in vegetables, fruits, whole grains, nuts, legumes, and seafood, while limiting sugar-sweetened foods and beverages, refined grains, and processed meats. When one follows this dietary pattern routinely over the course of time, the risk of age-related cognitive decline appears to decrease.

Putting it all together

How you use these 10 lifestyle factors to help reduce your risk of developing Alzheimer's disease or other forms of dementia is up to you. To make a complete overhaul of your lifestyle overnight is unrealistic. Keep it simple. Focus on one or two factors to begin with, making them a part of your daily life while gradually adding in others over time. The key is to stick with these factors for the long run. It also helps to know that you have more control over your health than you may believe. But until you take steps to improve your health, you may never know the profound difference it can make.

CHAPTER EIGHT

RECIPES PROMOTING BRAIN HEALTH

"All my life I had been 'Daddy's girl.' He had such a positive influence on me and our relationship was strong throughout my life. He was always there for me, giving me guidance, support, and advice whenever I needed his fatherly help. When he was diagnosed with Alzheimer's, it was devastating for our family. The Daddy I once knew was suddenly replaced by someone I no longer recognized. I remember one day eating lunch with my parents. Out of the blue, my Daddy suddenly looked at me, said he didn't know who I was, wanted me to leave and to get out of his house. I went back to work feeling crushed and cried for hours. My 'old' Daddy would have never said that to me in a million years."

-Daresa
Daughter of Humbert, who was diagnosed
with Alzheimer's disease at the age of 79.

The goal of this book has been to provide you with information supported by scientific evidence regarding how certain nutrients and foods promote brain health. The recipes that follow in this chapter are simple, delicious and brain-healthy. Most of us prefer recipes that are easy to follow, don't require precooking or hard-to-find ingredients or anything that is not doable as a weeknight meal. I hope you find the following recipes to fit that bill and enjoy them as much as I have.

Baked Oatmeal with Berries and Lentils

Rise and shine for lentils. Lentils? Of course! The combo of lentils and oats is perfect for stabilizing cholesterol levels making it both heart and brain friendly. Impress your family or guests with this simple oatmeal with berries for an easy, hearty breakfast. They'll know lentils are part of the mix for added protein and fiber.

Brain-boosting ingredients: **lentils, oats, and berries**

Brain-boosting nutrients: **protein, folate, and fiber**

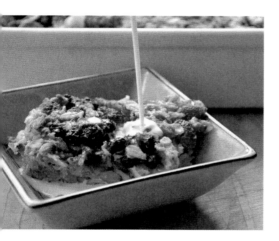

INGREDIENTS:

- 1 ½ cup old-fashioned rolled oats
- ¼ cup red lentils
- 1 teaspoon baking powder
- 1 teaspoon cinnamon
- ¼ teaspoon salt or sea salt
- 1 cup fresh or frozen blueberries, raspberries, or both
- 1/3 cup shredded coconut (optional)
- 2 cups milk
- 1/3 cup maple syrup
- 1 large egg
- 2 tablespoon butter, melted and cooked slightly
- 2 teaspoons vanilla extract

1. Preheat oven to 375 degrees F.

2. In an 8-inch square baking dish, mix together the oats, lentils, baking powder, cinnamon, and salt. Scatter with berries and coconut.

3. In another bowl, whisk together the milk, maple syrup, egg, butter, and vanilla. Pour the mixture over the oats, and give it a gentle stir to distribute everything evenly.

4. Bake for 40 minutes, or until the to is golden and the oats have set. Serve warm, topped with milk or a splash of cream. Leftovers reheat beautifully.

Nutrition: 180 calories, 7 g total fat, 3.5 g saturated fat, 6 g protein, 25 g carbohydrate, 3 g fiber. Servings – 8; Serving size: 1 cup

Recipe courtesy of www.lentils.org

Veggie Scrambled Eggs with Cheese

Looking for something different besides cold cereal or toast? Here's a breakfast that has it all – protein, veggies and a side of fruit. This quick, easy, and filling start to your day is a delicious way to nourish your brain. Breakfast can be a difficult meal to get in veggies but this recipe makes it super easy.

Brain-boosting ingredients: **eggs and veggies**

Brain-boosting nutrients: **protein, vitamins A and C, antioxidants and fiber**

INGREDIENTS:

- 2 tablespoons butter
- 5 eggs
- Salt and pepper to taste
- 2 cups washed baby spinach, chopped
- 3 green onions, thinly sliced, both green and white part
- 12 cherry tomatoes, halved or quartered
- 2 tablespoons chopped basil
- ½ cup grated cheese – your choice

1. Preheat skillet over medium-high heat and add butter to melt.

2. Whisk eggs together in a bowl, season with salt and pepper.

3. Add spinach and green onion to preheated skillet. Sauté until spinach is slightly wilted, less than 1 minutes.

4. Add egg mixture to pan, stir constantly. When eggs are almost set, add cherry tomatoes, basil and cheese. Continue to stir constantly to mix ingredients.

5. When eggs are set, remove from pan, garnish with additional shredded cheese and serve immediately.

Nutrition: 138 calories, 10 g total fat, 4 g saturated fat, 10 g protein, 2 g carbohydrate, 2 g fiber.
Servings – 2; Serving size: 1 cup

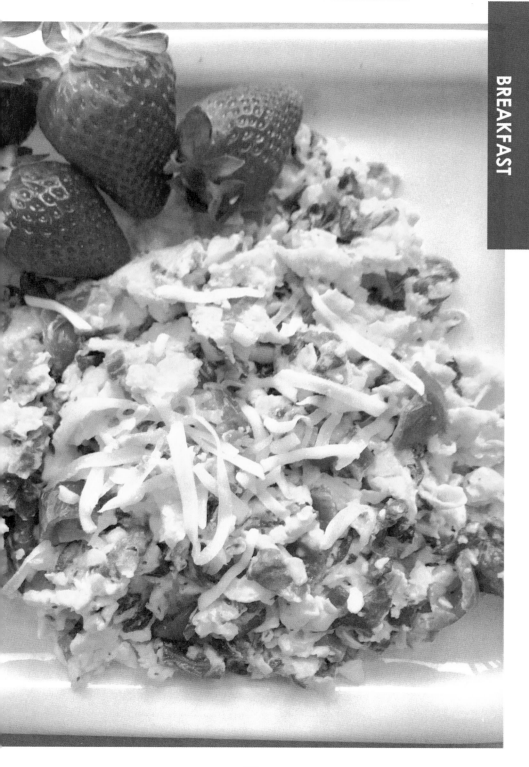

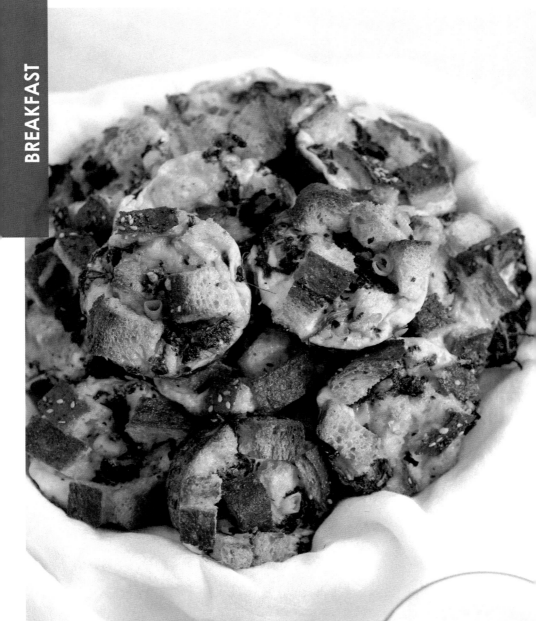

*Nutrition: 258 calories, 14 g total fat, 5 g saturated fat,
16 g protein, 17 g carbohydrate, 4 g fiber.
Servings – 12; Serving size: 1 muffin tin-size casserole*

Grab and Go Mini Breakfast Casseroles

Looking for a protein-packed, grab and go breakfast without having to resort to a high-protein drink concoction? This is your answer. Make during the weekend, then refrigerate (up to 3 days) or freeze and your "What will I have for breakfast?" worries are over for the majority of the week. Reheat in a toaster oven or microwave and you'll be out the door in no time. Pair two mini casseroles with 8 ounces of milk for a satisfying 24 grams of protein along with a handful of berries or an orange for a healthy dose of vitamin C to kick start your day.

Brain-boosting ingredients: **eggs, spinach, and side of berries**

Brain-boosting nutrients: protein, **vitamins A and C, fiber, and antioxidants**

BREAKFAST

INGREDIENTS:

- Canola or olive oil pan spray
- 4-5 slices whole-wheat bread, cubed
- 2 tablespoons extra-virgin olive oil
- 1 cup reduced-fat sharp Cheddar cheese, shredded
- 3 scallions, green parts sliced, white part chopped
- 1 teaspoon salt-free garlic and herb seasoning (or use ½ teaspoon garlic powder)
- ¼ teaspoon salt
- Freshly ground black pepper
- 1 (10-ounce) package frozen chopped spinach, thawed and water squeezed out well
- 5 large eggs
- 1 ¼ cups lowfat milk

1. Coat muffin tin with pan spray. Preheat oven to 375 degrees Fahrenheit.

2. In a large mixing bowl, coat cubed bread with olive oil. Add cheese, scallions, garlic seasoning, salt and pepper, and crumble in the spinach. Stir well. Divide bread mixture evenly among the 12 muffin tin wells.

3. In the same mixing bowl, beat the eggs and stir in milk. Pour the mixture over the bread in the muffin tin.

4. Bake for 30 minutes or until the bread on top is golden and crispy and the centers are set, not wet-looking. Or insert a toothpick into the center and it should come out clean.

5. Cool for 5 minutes. Cut around the edges of the casseroles to remove from the muffin tins. Leftovers can be reheated in the toaster oven or microwave.

Recipe from www.milklife.com

Brain-Boosting Berry Smoothie

Word has it that powerful antioxidants and phytochemicals in berries may improve cognitive function. When paired with omega-3 rich walnuts, it's a berry smoothie match made in heaven. This tasty smoothie will work its magic on your memory so try this unforgettable brain cell-supporting smoothie.

Brain-boosting ingredients: **blueberries, raspberries, and walnuts**

Brain-boosting nutrients: **vitamins A and C , Omega-3 fatty acids, antioxidants, and fiber**

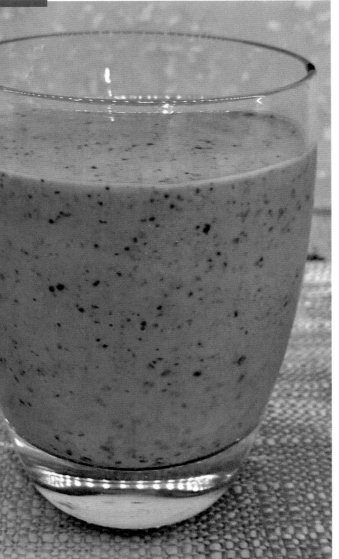

INGREDIENTS:
- ½ cup orange juice
- 1 cup plain Greek yogurt
- 1 ½ cups frozen blueberries
- ½ cup frozen raspberries
- 1-2 tablespoons chia seeds
- ¼ cup walnuts

1. Combine the orange juice and yogurt in a blender. Add the blueberries, raspberries, chia seeds, and walnuts. Blend until smooth.

Nutrition: 180 calories, 2 g total fat, 0 g saturated fat, 10 g protein, 30 g carbohydrate, 5 g fiber. Servings – 2 ; Serving size – 1 ¼ cups

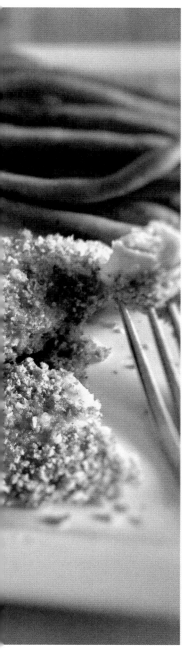

Walnut Crusted Chicken Breast Tenders

Who would guess that chicken and walnuts is quite the nutrition-powered combo. Poultry provides high-quality protein as well as iron, zinc, and vitamin B12 essential for brain health. Walnuts are packed with omega-3 fatty acids, giving both a brain and heart boost. The walnut-based coating adds richness to this light breading keeping the chicken moist and delicious.

Brain-boosting foods – chicken, walnuts, and 100% whole wheat bread

Brain-boosting nutrients – iron, zinc, vitamin B12, omega-3 fatty acids, fiber, and protein

INGREDIENTS:

- 2 slices 100% whole-wheat bread, dried
- ½ cup walnuts
- 2 tablespoons Parmesan cheese
- 2 eggs
- About 1 pound chicken breast tenders
- 1 teaspoon salt
- ½ teaspoon black pepper

1. Preheat oven to 350 degrees Fahrenheit.

2. In a food processor or blender, combine bread, walnuts, Parmesan cheese, salt and pepper. Process until fine breadcrumbs form. Transfer to a shallow bowl.

3. Beat eggs in a separate shallow bowl until mixed

4. Dip each chicken tender into egg mixture, let excess drip off, and then dip into crumb mixture, covering tenders completely.

5. Place tenders side-by-side in a baking dish sprayed with cooking oil. Place in oven and bake for approximately 45 minutes.

Nutrition: 375 calories, 23 g total fat, 5 g saturated fat, 28 g protein, 14 g carbohydrate, 2.5 g fiber.
Servings 4; Serving size – 3 ounces

LUNCH AND DINNER

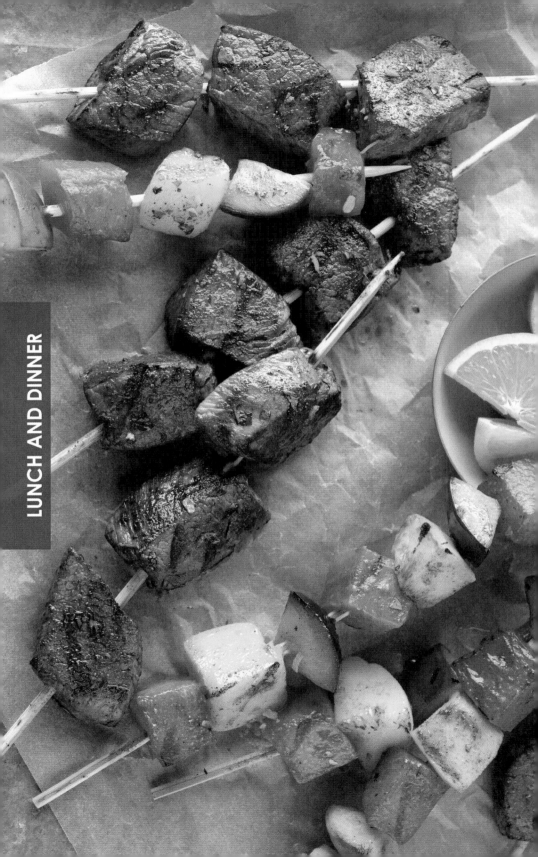

Citrus Marinated Beef Top Sirloin & Fruit Kabobs

Made with lean beef, this recipe is a for-sure crowd pleaser. This is good eating with a twist – mixing beef with fruit. Low in total and saturated fat, rich in iron, zinc, and vitamin B 12, your family will want you to make it again and again.

Brain-boosting foods – **lean beef, peppers, and fruit**

Brain-boosting nutrients – **iron, zinc, vitamin B12, protein, niacin, fiber, vitamins A and C, and antioxidants**

INGREDIENTS:

- 1 beef Top Sirloin Steak Center Cut, Boneless (about 1 pound)
- 1 medium orange
- ¼ cup fresh cilantro, chopped
- 1 tablespoon smoked paprika
- ¼ teaspoon ground red pepper (optional)
- 4 cups mango, watermelon, peaches, and/or plums, cubed

1. Grate, peel, and squeeze 2 tablespoons juice from orange; reserve juice. Combine orange peel, cilantro, paprika, and ground red pepper, if desired, in small bowl. Cut beef steak into 1 1/4–inch pieces. Place beef and 2 ½ tablespoons cilantro mixture in food-safe plastic bag; turn to coat. Place remaining cilantro mixture and fruit in separate food-safe plastic bag; turn to coat. Close bags securely. Marinate beef and fruit in refrigerator 15 minutes to 2 hours.

2. Soak eight 9-inch bamboo skewers in water for 10 minutes. Thread beef evenly onto four skewers leaving small space between pieces. Thread fruit onto remaining four separate skewers.

3. Place kabobs on grill over medium, ash-covered coals. Grill beef kabobs, covered, 5 to 7 minutes (over medium heat on preheated gas grill 7 to 8 minutes) for medium rare (145 degrees Fahrenheit) to medium (160 degrees Fahrenheit) doneness, turning occasionally. Grill fruit kabobs 5 to 7 minutes or until softened and beginning to brown, turning once.

4. Drizzle reserved orange juice over fruit kabobs. Garnish with cilantro, if desired.

Nutrition: 239 calories, 5.7 g total fat, 1.8 g saturated fat, 28 g protein, 22 g carbohydrate, 3.4 g fiber. Servings 4; Serving size – 1 skewer steak and 1 skewer fruit

Recipe courtesy of www.beefitswhatsfordinner.com

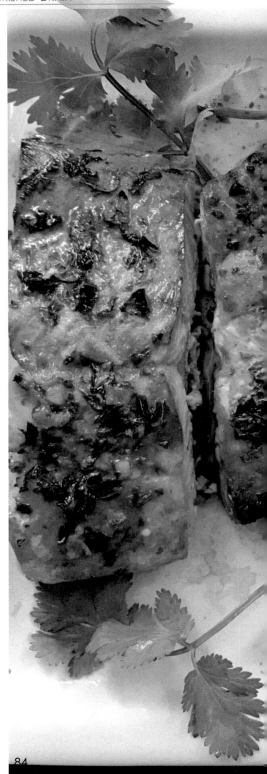

Mediterranean Salmon

For anyone who may be intimidated to cook fish, here is a fearless recipe making it super easy. Not only will you be fixing a delicious, gourmet meal but it's a dinner that can be on your table in just 20 minutes. As you eat this flavor-filled salmon, you can also enjoy knowing you're getting a great source of monounsaturated fat and brain-boosting omega-3 fatty acids.

Brain-boosting food –
salmon and olive oil

Brain-boosting nutrients –
**omega-3 fatty acids, protein,
monounsaturated fat,
vitamin B12, potassium, and
antioxidants**

INGREDIENTS:
- ½ cup olive oil
- ¼ cup balsamic vinegar
- 4 cloves garlic, pressed
- 4 3-ounce salmon fillets
- 1 tablespoon fresh cilantro, chopped
- 1 tablespoon fresh basil, chopped
- 1 ½ teaspoon garlic salt

LUNCH AND DINNER

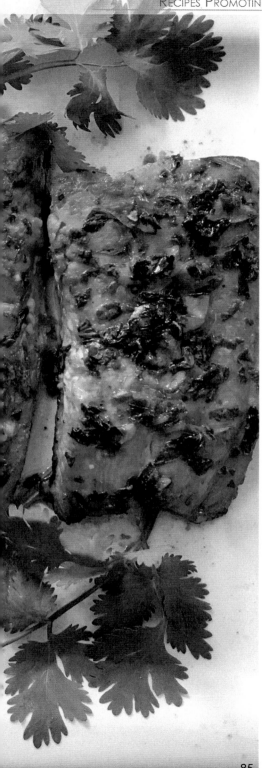

1. Mix together olive oil and balsamic vinegar in a small bowl.

2. Arrange salmon fillets in a shallow baking dish. Rub pressed garlic onto the fillets, then pour the vinegar and oil over them, turning once to coat.

3. Season with cilantro, basil, and garlic salt. Set aside to marinate for 10 minutes.

4. Preheat oven's broiler. Place the salmon about 6 inches from the heat source and broil for 15 minutes, turning once or until browned on both sides and easily flaked with a fork.

5. Brush occasionally with the sauce from the pan.

LUNCH AND DINNER

Nutrition: 236 calories, 12 g total fat, 4 g saturated fat, 30 g protein, 2 g carbohydrate, 1 g fiber. Servings – 4; Serving size – 3-4 ounce fillets

Recipe courtesy of Dr. David B. Samadi, Urologic Oncologist Expert and Renowned Robotic Surgeon
www.samadimd.com
www.prostatecancer911.com
www.roboticoncology.com

Easy Salmon/Tuna Cakes

How many times do you wish you had an idea for a simple, quick and healthy meal that takes less than 10 minutes to make? Here it is. This very tasty, easy-to-put together recipe is chock full of nutrients not only promoting brain health but also heart, skin, and nail health too. Use either salmon or tuna, whichever you prefer.

Brain-boosting foods – **salmon or tuna, egg, and peppers**

Brain-boosting nutrients – **omega-3 fatty acids, protein, vitamin B12, selenium, potassium, vitamins A and C**

INGREDIENTS:

- 2 6-ounce cans or pouches of salmon or tuna
- 2 eggs, beaten
- 1/2 cup onion, finely diced
- 1/2 cup bell peppers, green or red, finely diced
- 2 teaspoons lemon juice
- ½ teaspoon salt
- ½ teaspoon pepper
- 6-8 tablespoons bread crumbs (bought or homemade)
- 4 teaspoons olive oil

1. Mix together salmon or tuna with beaten egg, diced onions and diced bell peppers.

2. Season with salt, pepper and lemon juice.

3. Mix in 2 tablespoons bread crumbs

4. Form into patties, coating patties with additional bread crumbs

5. Heat olive oil in a pan or skillet over medium-high heat.

6. Place patties in oil, turning over once and cook until both sides are brown and crispy.

Nutrition: 180 calories, 10 g total fat, 2 g saturated fat, 20 g protein, 2 g carbohydrate, 1 g fiber. Servings – 4; Serving size – 3 ounces

LUNCH AND DINNER

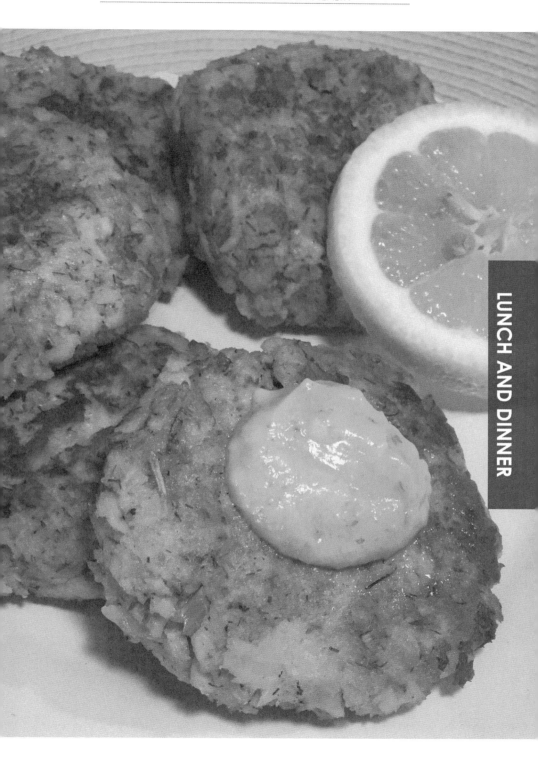

Vegetarian Vegetable Pasta Primavera

Oohh la la! This absolutely delicious and nutritious meal is a winner, perfect for a light lunch or dinner. Whole wheat pasta is suggested as the base for the veggies as it provides an extra dose of fiber, phosphorus, magnesium, and folate.

Brain-boosting foods – **whole wheat pasta, various veggies, and olive oil**

Brain-boosting nutrients – **vitamins A, C, E, and K, omega-3 fatty acids, fiber, folate, magnesium, beta carotene, and lutein**

INGREDIENTS:

- 8-ounces whole wheat pasta – spaghetti, rotini, or bowtie – your choice
- 1 cup each of cut bite sized pieces of broccoli, cauliflower, carrots, and peas
- 1 cup fresh tomato, cut into chunks
- 2-4 teaspoons olive oil
- 2 teaspoons red wine vinegar
- 2 teaspoons lemon juice
- 1-2 tablespoons of fresh basil, chopped
- Parmesan cheese, if desired

LUNCH AND DINNER

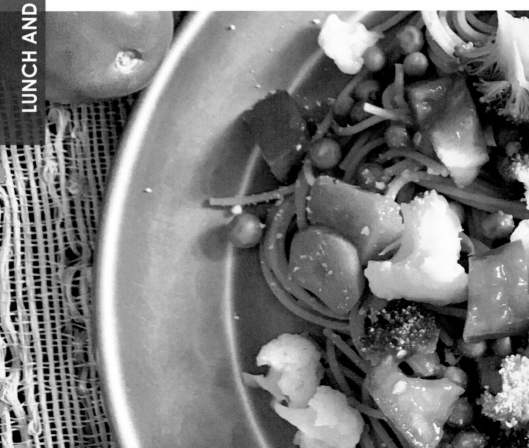

1. Follow directions for cooking whole grain pasta

2. Cut up broccoli, cauliflower, carrots, and peas. Bring a large saucepan of salted water to a boil, add in all vegetables except for the tomato, cooking for about 5 minutes or until crisp tender.

3. Drain vegetables into a colander

4. While vegetables and pasta are cooking, prepare olive oil dressing by mixing together the olive oil, red wine vinegar and lemon juice.

5. Drain pasta and vegetables into separate colanders.

6. Place pasta on a plate, spoon cooked vegetables over the pasta, then add in chunks of tomato and chopped fresh basil.

7. Drizzle each plate of pasta and vegetables with olive oil dressing.

8. If desired, sprinkle with Parmesan cheese.

Nutrition: 252 calories, 4.5 g total fat, 0 g saturated fat, 8 g protein, 45 g carbohydrate, 12 g fiber. Servings – 4; Serving size – ½ cup pasta and ½ cup vegetables

LUNCH AND DINNER

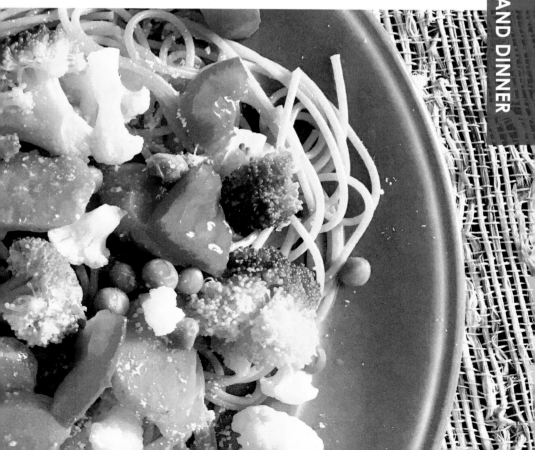

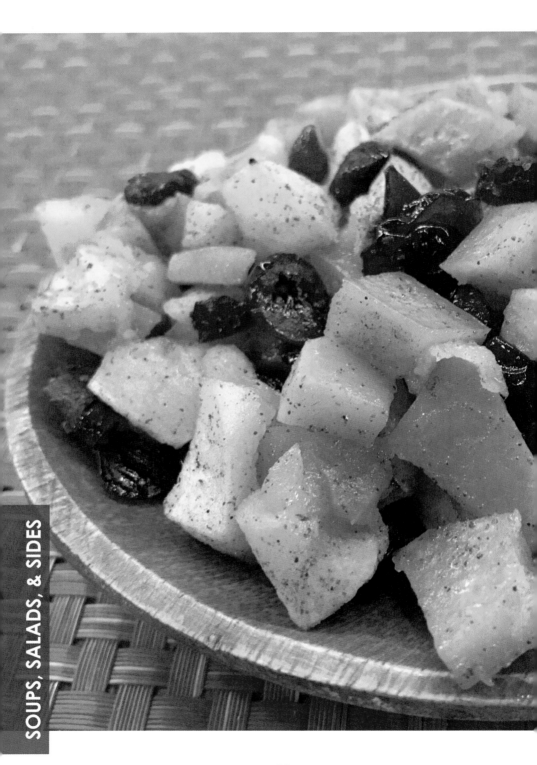

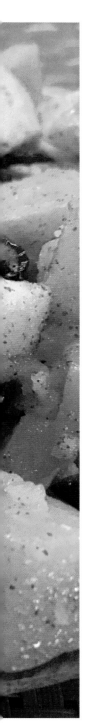

Baked Butternut Squash with Apples & Cranberries

This hearty and healthy recipe has all the warmth of fall wrapped into this one seasonably delicious dish. If you don't care for butternut squash, you can substitute it with acorn or buttercup squash. If dried cranberries are not a favorite, use raisins or dried cherries or leave out altogether. Use apples meant for baking such as Granny Smith, Honeycrisp, Jonathans, Winesap, Braeburn, or Rome Beauty.

Brain-boosting foods: **squash, apples, and dried fruit**

Brain-boosting nutrients: **vitamin A, C and K, magnesium, potassium, phosphorous, fiber, beta carotene, and lutein**

INGREDIENTS:

- 2 cups squash cubes
- 2 cups apple cubes
- 1 tablespoon olive oil or canola oil
- ½ teaspoon ground cinnamon
- ½ teaspoon ground nutmeg
- 1 tablespoon sugar
- ½ teaspoon salt

1. Preheat oven to 425 degrees Fahrenheit.

2. Peel the squash and apples cutting into bite sized pieces or cubes.

3. Combine squash and apple pieces, oil, cinnamon, nutmeg, sugar, and salt in a large bowl.

4. Toss to coat squash and apples evenly.

5. Spread mixture on a metal baking pan.

6. Bake in oven for 20 to 30 minutes or until squash is soft.

Nutrition: 164 calories, 4 g total fat, 0.5 g saturated fat, 2 g protein, 30 g carbohydrate, 5 g fiber. Servings – 4; Serving size – ½ cup

SOUPS, SALADS, & SIDES

Lemon Broccoli with Dried Cherries Salad

Needing a go-to side dish from upcoming summer gatherings to stay-at-home family meals? This recipe fits the bill. From the tantalizing tangy dressing to the hint of sweetness from the cherries, this salad will be a favorite.

Brain-boosting foods: **broccoli, olive oil, and cherries**

Brain-boosting nutrients: **vitamins, A, C, and K, omega-3 fatty acids, fiber, folate, magnesium, beta carotene, and lutein**

INGREDIENTS:

- 1 large head of broccoli, cut into florets, stems peeled and sliced ½ inch
- ¼ cup extra-virgin olive oil
- 2 tablespoons red wine vinegar
- ½ tablespoons fresh lemon juice
- 1 teaspoon lemon zest, finely grated
- ½ of a small shallot, minced
- ½ cup dried cherries
- Kosher salt and ground black pepper

1. Fill a large saucepan with salted water and bring to a boil.

2. Add broccoli florets and cook for about 5 minutes or until bright green and tender. Drain into a colander and rinse with cold water; pat dry.

3. In a large bowl, whisk olive oil with the vinegar, lemon juice, lemon zest, shallot, and dried cherries. Season with salt and pepper to taste.

4. Add the broccoli, toss to coat and serve.

Nutrition: 162 calories, 6 g total fat, 0.5 g saturated fat, 2 g protein, 25 g carbohydrate, 6 g fiber. Servings – 4; Serving size – ½ cup

SOUPS, SALADS, & SIDES

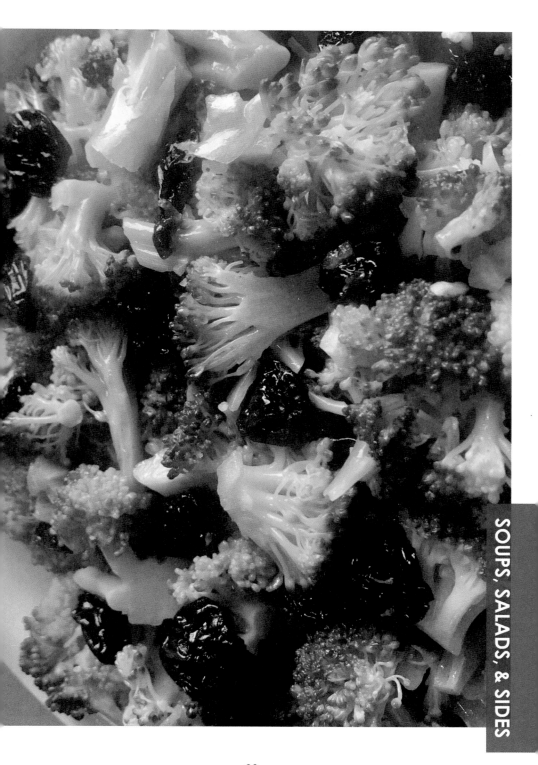

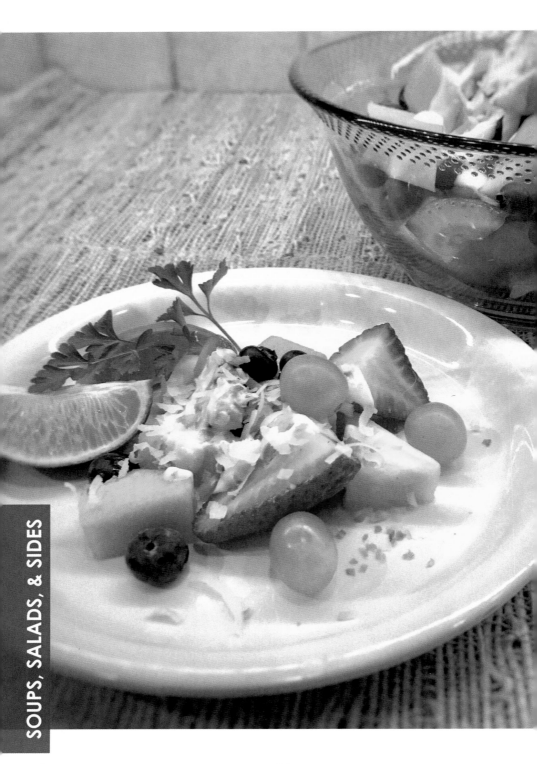

SOUPS, SALADS, & SIDES

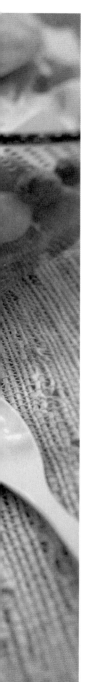

Creamy Key Lime Fruit Salad

A perfect dish to "wow and impress your summer guests," this salad can do the same year-round. From the "pop" of color to the nice blend of summer fruit with key lime yogurt (or try vanilla yogurt and call it "Creamy Vanilla Fruit Salad"), topped with crunchy toasted coconut…it's incredibly good!

Brain-boosting foods: **Fruit**

Brain-boosting nutrients: **vitamins A, C, E, and K, fiber, flavonoid, antioxidants, beta carotene, lutein, and zeaxanthin**

INGREDIENTS:

- 2 6-ounce Key lime pie-flavored yogurt
- 4 tablespoons of freshly squeezed orange juice
- 2 cups fresh pineapple chunks
- 1 cup strawberry halves
- 2 cups green grapes, halved or whole
- 1 cup blueberries
- 2 cups cantaloupe, cubed
- ¼ cup flaked or shredded coconut, toasted

1. Heat a skillet over medium-low heat. Add coconut stirring frequently for 6-12 minutes stir constantly until golden brown.

2. Mix yogurt and juice

3. Layer food in order listed above in 2-½ quart clear glass bowl.

4. Pour yogurt mixture over fruit and sprinkle with coconut. Serve immediately.

Nutrition: 130 calories, 2 g total fat, 1 g saturated fat, 2 g protein, 26 g carbohydrate, 3 g fiber. Servings – 8; Serving size – ½ cup

SOUPS, SALADS, & SIDES

Tomato Veggie Split Pea Soup

When the weather turns cold, nothing sounds better than steaming hot homemade soup! When each spoonful is loaded with veggies, it makes it even better. This wholesome, hearty vegetarian meal has great texture and taste and when paired with crusty bread, it's a match made in heaven.

Brain-boosting foods: **each veggie in the recipe and split peas**

Brain-boosting nutrients: **fiber, vitamins A, C, E, and K, lutein, zeaxanthin, fiber, potassium, protein, and antioxidants**

INGREDIENTS:

- 1 tablespoon olive oil
- ½ of a large onion, finely chopped
- 1 stalk celery, diced
- 2 cloves garlic, finely minced
- 2 large carrots, chopped
- 1 cup frozen corn
- 1 can (14.5 ounce) black beans
- ½ medium zucchini, chopped
- 2 cubes chicken bouillon
- 1 teaspoon dried thyme leaves
- ¼ teaspoon black pepper
- 2 cans (14.5 ounce) petite diced tomatoes, undrained
- 1 cup dried green split peas
- 4 cups water

1. Heat oil in 3-quart saucepan over medium heat. Cook onion, celery, and garlic in oil about 5 minutes until softened.

2. Stir in remaining ingredients. Heat to boiling, then reduce heat. Cover and simmer about 20-30 minutes or until heated through.

Nutrition: 190 calories, 2 g total fat, 1 g saturated fat, 13 g protein, 30 g carbohydrate, 12 g fiber. Servings – 8; Serving size – ½ cup

SOUPS, SALADS, & SIDES

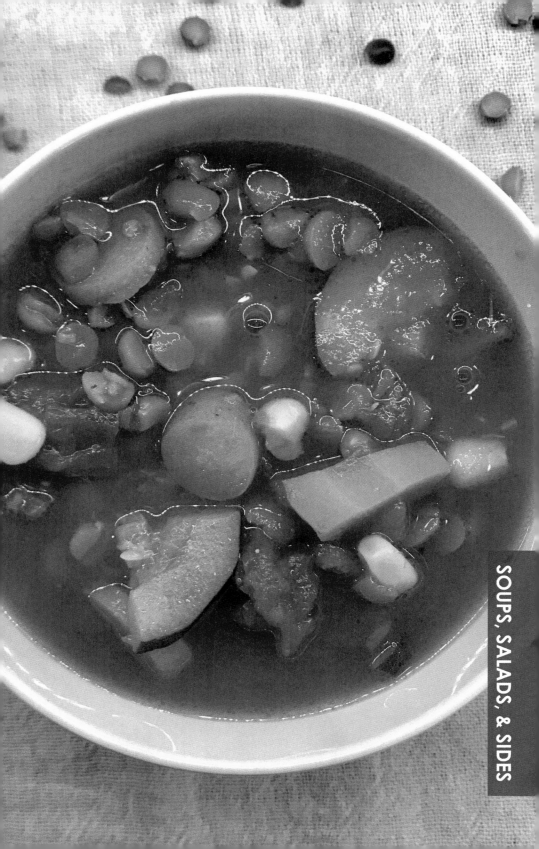

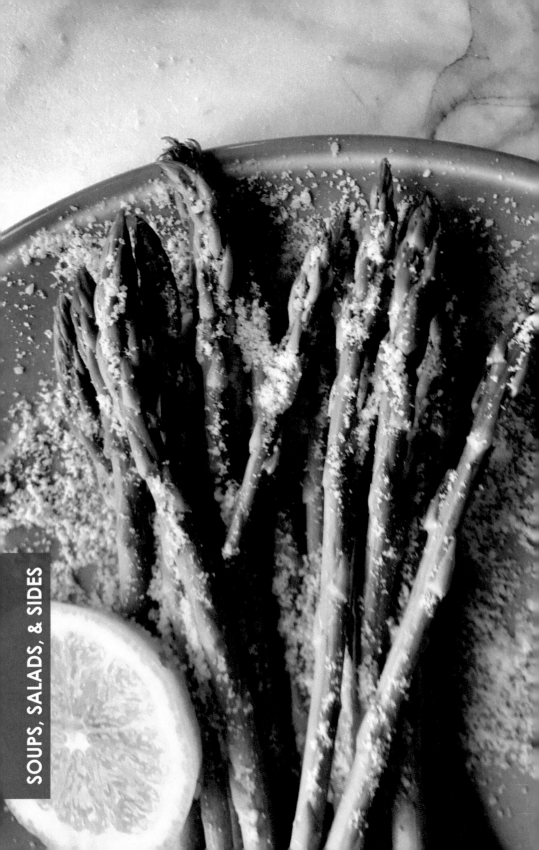

SOUPS, SALADS, & SIDES

Oven Roasted Lemon Parmesan Asparagus

A springtime favorite, one of the best ways to cook asparagus is to roast it in the oven. Roasting strong-tasting vegetables like asparagus helps to caramelize the flavor and reduce the natural bitterness they have. Even the pickiest of eaters will find a liking to roasted asparagus.

Brain-boosting food: asparagus and olive oil

Brain-boosting nutrients: fiber, folate, vitamins A, C, E, and K, lutein, antioxidants, monounsaturated fat, and omega-3 fatty acids

INGREDIENTS:

- 1 bunch of asparagus spears
- 3 tablespoons olive oil
- 1 tablespoon Parmesan cheese
- 1 clove garlic, chopped
- 1 teaspoon salt
- ½ teaspoon pepper
- 1 tablespoon fresh lemon juice

1. Preheat oven to 425 degrees Fahrenheit.

2. Wash and trim asparagus.

3. Place asparagus in a single layer on a baking sheet. Drizzle olive oil over spears, then toss spears to coat.

4. Sprinkle 1 tablespoon of Parmesan cheese over spears

5. Distribute chopped garlic evenly over spears.

6. Sprinkle salt and pepper evenly over spears.

7. Drizzle fresh lemon juice over spears.

8. Bake until tender, 12-15 minutes.

Nutrition: 113 calories, 5 g total fat, 0.5 g saturated fat, 2 g protein, 15 g carbohydrate, 3 g fiber. Servings – 4; Serving size – 1 cup

SOUPS, SALADS, & SIDES

Chia Seed Blueberry Banana Muffins

Moist, not too sweet, a nice blend of two fruits, and an interesting "crunch" courtesy of the chia seeds, this muffin has it all. Better yet, it provides several brain-boosting nutrients making this muffin a nutrient dense addition to any meal or snack.

Brain-boosting foods: **blueberries, banana, chia seeds, and whole wheat flour**

Brain-boosting nutrients: **omega-3 fatty acids, protein, fiber, vitamin C, fiber, lutein, and antioxidants**

INGREDIENTS:
- ½ cup canola oil
- 1 egg
- ¼ cup sugar
- 1 banana
- 1 ½ cups whole wheat flour
- 1 teaspoon baking soda
- ¼ teaspoon salt
- 1 teaspoon cinnamon
- 1 ½ teaspoon nutmeg
- 2 tablespoons chia seeds
- ½ to ¾ cup blueberries (frozen or fresh)
- 1 teaspoon vanilla

1. Preheat oven to 375 degrees Fahrenheit.
2. Mix oil, egg and sugar in a large mixing bowl until smooth; add in banana mixing well.
3. Blend the dry ingredients well in a separate bowl – flour, baking soda, salt, cinnamon, nutmeg, and chia seeds
4. Add dry ingredients to oil mixture. Add in blueberries and Vanilla. Gently stir together just until moistened – do not overmix.
5. Spoon batter into muffin tin tray sprayed with vegetable pan spray.
6. Bake 15 to 20 minutes.

Nutrition: 135 calories, 3 g total fat, 1.5 g saturated fat, 2 g protein, 25 g carbohydrate, 4 g fiber. Servings – 12 muffins; Serving size – 1 muffin

SOUPS, SALADS, & SIDES

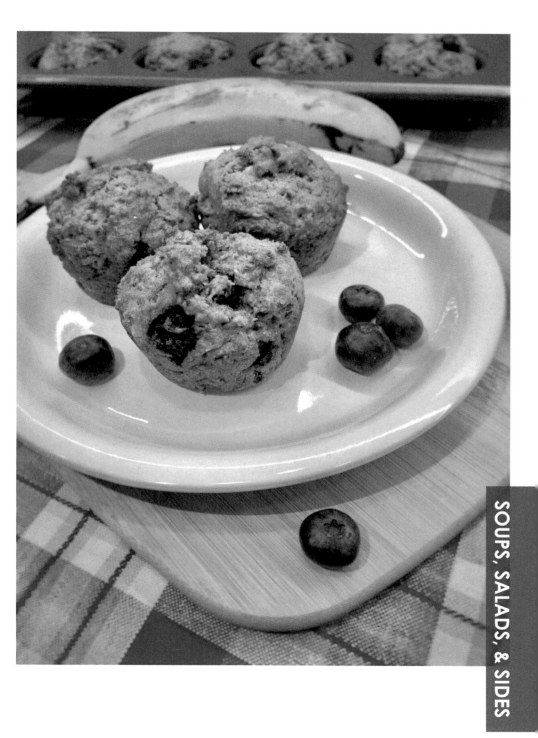

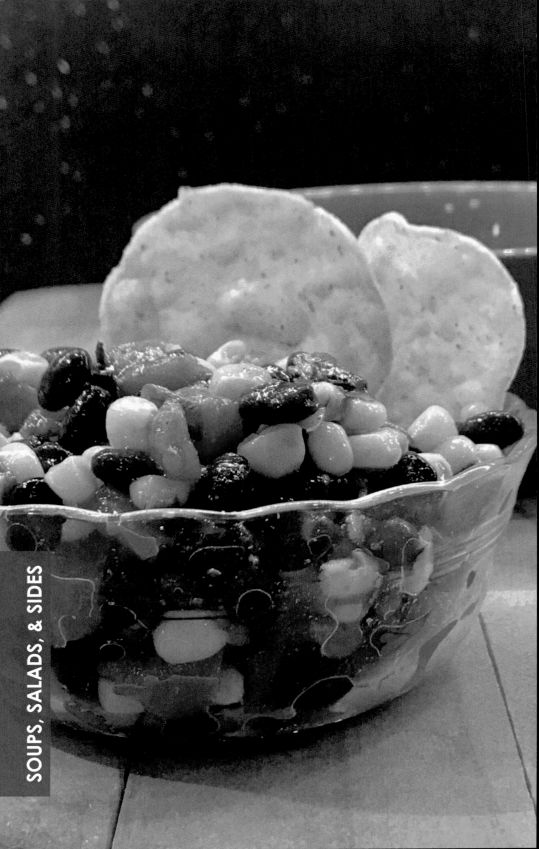

Black Bean and Corn Salsa

This salsa always receives rave reviews. Whether you use it for chips, pita bread or over grilled meat, it's simple to assemble, healthy, and best of all, tastes great.

Brain-boosting foods: **black beans, corn, and tomatoes**

Brain-boosting nutrients: **fiber, protein, antioxidants, vitamin C, and lutein**

INGREDIENTS:

- 1 (15-ounce can) black beans, drained and rinsed
- 1 (11-ounce can) whole kernel corn, drained
- 1 (14.5-ounce can) petite diced tomatoes, drained
- ½ cup green onions, chopped
- 2 tablespoons fresh cilantro, chopped
- ½ cup Italian salad dressing
- 2 serrano chiles, seeded, chopped (optional)

1. Combine all ingredients together in a large bowl, mixing well.

2. Refrigerate until serving

Nutrition: 144 calories, 8 g total fat, 2 g saturated fat, 4 g protein, 14 g carbohydrate, 4 g fiber.
Servings – 4 cups or 8 servings; Serving size – ½ cup

SOUPS, SALADS, & SIDES

Tropical Mango Guacamole

Shake up your tired old "guac" with this recipe. Take your classic guacamole out for a spin by adding in a couple of unusual ingredients – mango and jicama. Trust me, you won't be sorry.

Brain-boosting foods: **mango, avocado, and red pomegranate seeds**

Brain-boosting nutrients: **vitamins A, C, and E, omega-3 fatty acids, monounsaturated fat, fiber, and protein**

INGREDIENTS:

- 1 ripe mango, diced into ¼-inch cubes
- ¼ cup jicama, diced into ¼-inch cubes
- ¼ cup red onion, finely chopped
- ¼ cup garlic, finely chopped
- 2 tablespoons fresh lemon juice
- ½ teaspoon salt
- ¼ teaspoon black pepper
- 2 ripe avocados, peeled
- 2 tablespoons cilantro, chopped
- 1 tablespoon red pomegranate seeds (optional for garnish)

1. In a medium size bowl, mix the mango, jicama, onion, garlic, lemon juice, salt, and black pepper. Set aside.
2. In another bowl, add the peeled avocado and mash until soft.
3. Add the mango mixture to the avocado and mix.
4. Top with cilantro and pomegranate seeds

Nutrition: 251 calories, 15 g total fat, 2 g saturated fat, 3 g protein, 26 g carbohydrate, 9 g fiber. Servings – 8; Serving size – ½ cup.

Recipe courtesy of The National Mango Board

SOUPS, SALADS, & SIDES

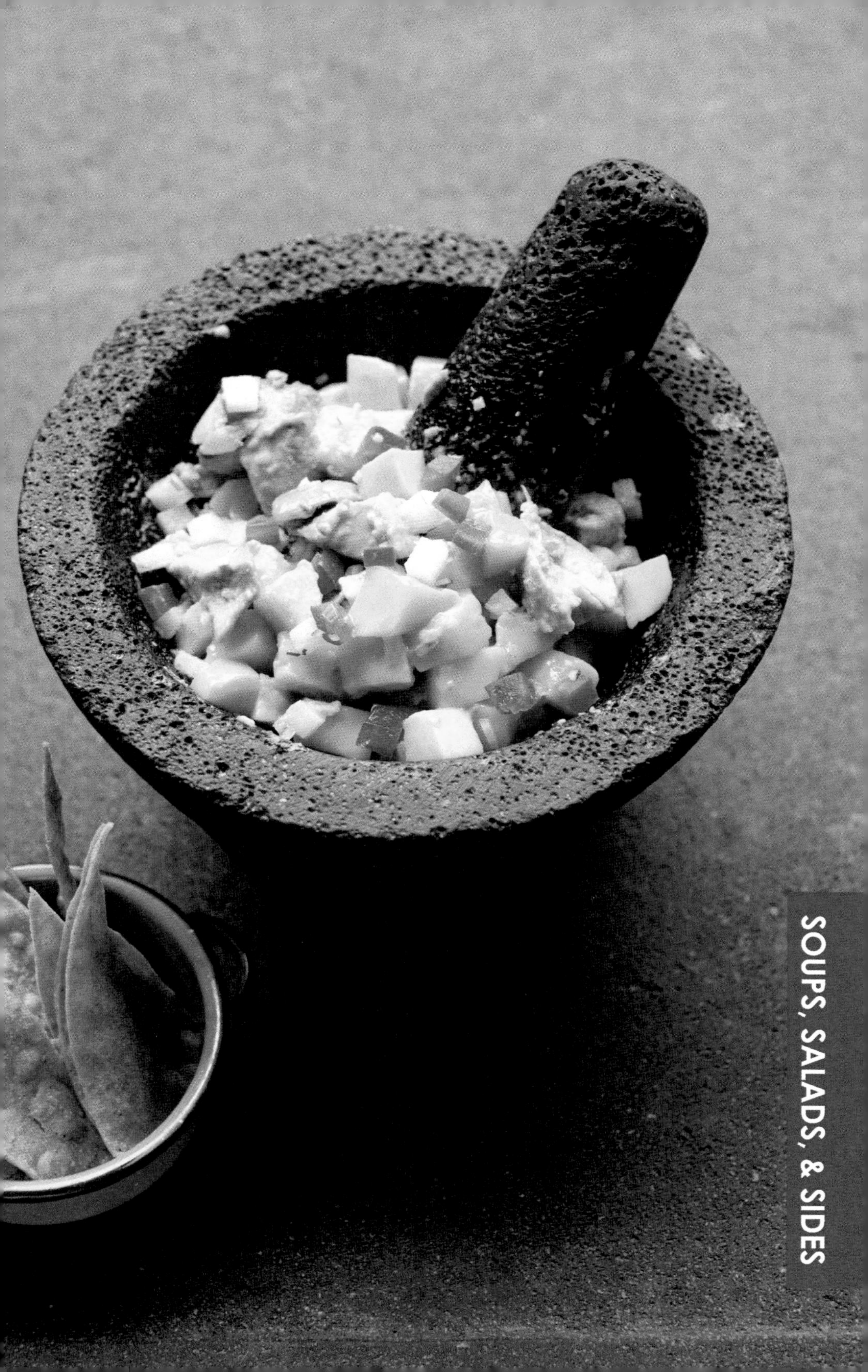

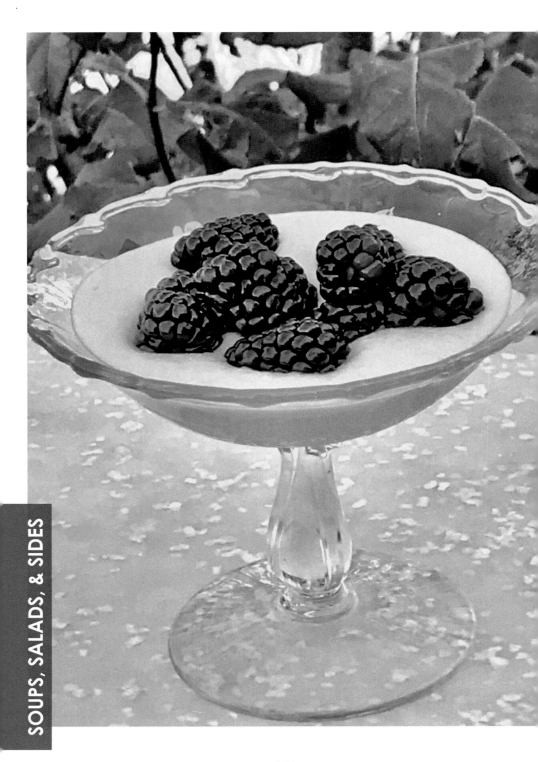

Blackberries with Sweet Almond Cashew Cream

Blackberries with cream are a culinary delight. Blackberries combined with a sweet cream offering less sugar and a healthier source of fat is perfection. You will come back to this pleasantly surprising recipe again and again, guaranteed. If blackberries are not your thing, this sweet cream also pairs well with fresh blueberries, strawberries, or freshly sliced peaches.

Brain-boosting foods: **berries and cashews**

Brain-boosting nutrients: **vitamins C and K, fiber, manganese, and antioxidants, and monounsaturated fat**

INGREDIENTS:

- 1 cup cashews
- 3 tablespoon maple syrup
- ¼ to ½ cup unsweetened vanilla almond milk
- 2 tablespoon lemon juice
- Pinch of salt
- ½ teaspoon vanilla extract
- Blackberries or other fresh fruit of your choice

1. Place cashews in a medium bowl, cover with hot water and soak for 30 minutes.
2. Drain cashews. Add cashews to a food processor along with the rest of the ingredients, except berries. Blend together until smooth.
3. Serve berries with cream.
4. Store cream in a jar in the refrigerator up to 3-4 days.

Nutrition: 170 calories, 6 g total fat, 1 g saturated fat, 3 g protein, 26 g carbohydrate, 4 g fiber. Servings – 4; Serving size – ¼ cup.

SOUPS, SALADS, & SIDES

ACKNOWLEDGMENTS

Writing this book would not have been possible without the support, encouragement, and guidance of so many influential people in my career and in my life. Five years ago, I never would have even considered such a venture but circumstances as they may be, led me down this path. My interest in writing began decades ago with my first job working as a WIC (Women, Infants, and Children) Dietitian when I began a monthly newsletter called the WIC Express at the Lyon County Health Department in Emporia, Kansas. Thanks to the administrator at that time, Eileen Greisher, I was allowed to write short articles on healthy eating for pregnancy, breastfeeding, and infants and childhood feeding along with recipes to educate our clients. This provided me a taste of the world of journalism and the need for a dietitian's expertise in nutrition.

I am also greatly indebted to the Osage County Online newspaper editor, Wayne White, who gave me the go-ahead to have my first regular nutrition column in his publication. Thanks to the Internet and various social media sources, this online exposure of my articles gave me more recognition than I ever would have imagined. One such source I am deeply grateful for is Dr. David B. Samadi, Urologic Oncologist Expert and World Renowned Robotic Surgeon at Lenox Hill Hospital in New York City. His willingness to take a chance and believe in me is very humbling.

I also want to acknowledge much thanks to my talented son, Peter, who spent tedious hours editing my book.

Most of all, I want to thank my family and my husband Casey for putting up with my long hours of work on this manuscript and for their constant encouragement and backing of this endeavor. If it wasn't for the loving support and patience of my family and colleagues at work cheering me on, this project may never have been completed. I thank each one of you.

REFERENCES

Chapter 1

1. 2018 Alzheimer's Disease, Facts and Figures

2. 2015 Alzheimer's Disease Facts and Figures. Alzheimer's Dement. 2015 Mar; 11(3):332-84.

3. Mortality Among Centenarians in the United States, 2000–2014: Centers for Disease Control and Prevention: Jiaquan Xu, M.D. 2016

Chapter 2

4. Potter, MC, Wyble, B, Hagmann, CE, et al. "Detecting meaning in RSVP at 13 ms per picture." *Attention, Perception, and Psychophysics* (2014) 76:270.

5. Wen-Juan Huang, Xia Zhang, and Wei-Wei Chen. "Role of oxidative stress in Alzheimer's disease." *Biomedical Reports*, (2016): 519-522.

Chapter 3

6. Morris MC, Tangney CC, Wang Y, Sacks FM, Bennett DA, Aggarwal NT. "MIND diet associated with reduced incidence of Alzheimer's disease." *Alzheimer's Dementia* (2015): 1007-1014.

7. Panagiotakos DB, Pitsavos C, Arvaniti F, Stefanadis C. "Adherence to the Mediterranean food pattern predicts the prevalence of hypertension, hypercholesterolemia, diabetes and obesity, among healthy adults; the accuracy of the MedDietScore." *Prev. Med*, (2007): 335-340.

8. Sacks FM, Appel LJ, Moore TJ, Obarzanek E, et al. "A dietary approach to prevent hypertension: a review of the Dietary Approaches to Stop Hypertension (DASH) Study." *Clinical Cardiology*, (1999): 1116-10.

9. Morris MC, Tangney CC, Wang Y, Sacks FM, Barnes LL, Bennett DA, Aggarwal NT. "MIND diet slows cognitive decline with aging." *Alzheimer's Dementia*, (2015): 1015-1022.

10. Tangney CC, Li H, Wang Y, Barnes L, Schneider JA, Bennett DA, Morris MC. "Relation of DASH-and Mediterranean-like dietary patterns to cognitive decline in older persons." *Neurology*, (2014): 1410-1416.

11. Wengreen H, Munger RG, Cutler A, Quach A, Bowles A, Corcoran C, Tschanz JT, et. al. "Prospective study of Dietary Approaches to Stop Hypertension-and Mediterranean-style dietary patterns and age-related cognitive change: the Cache County Study on Memory, Health and Aging." *American Journal of Clinical Nutrition*, (2013): 1263-1271.

12. Marcason, W. "What are the components to the MIND diet?" *Journal of the Academy of Nutrition and Dietetics,* (2015): 1744.

13. Shukitt-Hale B, Lau FC, Joseph JA. "Berry fruit supplementation and the aging brain." *Journal of Agricultural and Food Chemistry*, (2008): 636-641.

14. Perez L, Heim L, Sherzai A, Jaceldo-Siegl K, "Nutrition and vascular dementia." *The Journal of Nutrition, Health, and Aging*, (2012): 319-324.

15. Mohajeri MH, Troesch B, Weber P. "Inadequate supply of vitamins and DHA in the elderly: implication for brain aging and Alzheimer-type dementia." *Nutrition*, (2015): 261-275.

Chapter 4

16. Morris MS. "The role of B vitamins in preventing and treating cognitive impairment and decline." *Advanced Nutrition*, (2012): 801-812.

17. Haan MN, Miller JW, Aiello AE, Whitmer RA, et. al. "Homocysteine, B vitamins, and the incidence of dementia and cognitive impairment: results from the Sacramento Area Latino Study on Aging." *American Journal of Clinical Nutrition*, (2007): 511-517.

18. Institute of Medicine (US) Standing Committee on the Scientific Evaluation of Dietary Reference Intakes and its Panel on Folate, Other B vitamins, and Choline. "Dietary Reference Intakes for Thiamin, Riboflavin, Niacin, Vitamin B6, Folate, Vitamin B12, Pantothenic Acid, Biotin, and Choline." *National Academies Press*, (1998).

19. Luchsinger JA, Tang MX, Miller J, Green R, Mayeux R. "Relation of higher folate intake to lower risk of Alzheimer disease in the elderly." *Archives of Neurology*, (2007): 86-92.

20. Forbes SC, Holroyd-Leduc JM, Poulin MJ, Hogan DB. "Effect of nutrients, dietary supplements and vitamins on cognition: a systematic review and meta-analysis of randomized controlled trials." *Canadian Geriatrics Journal.* (2015): 231-245.

21. Durga J, van Boxtel MP, Schouten EG, Kok FJ, Jolles J, Katan MB, Verhoef P. "Effect of 3-year folic acid supplementation on cognitive function in older adults in the FACIT trial: a randomized, double blind, controlled trial. *Lancet*, (2007): 208-216.

22. Giorgio La Fata, Peter Weber, M. Hasan Mohajeri. "Effects of vitamin E on cognitive performance during ageing and in Alzheimer's disease. *Nutrients*, (2014): 5453-5472.

23. Johnson EJ, Vishwanathan R, Johnson MA, et. al. "Relationship between serum and brain carotenoids, alpha-tocopherol, and retinol concentrations and cognitive performance in the oldest old from the Georgia Centenarian Study." *Journal of Aging Research*, (2013): Published online.

24. Erdman JW, Smith JW, Kuchan MJ, Mohn ES, et. al. "Lutein and brain function." *Foods*, (2015): 547-564.

25. Macready AL, Kennedy OB, Ellis JA, Williams CM, Spencer JP, Butler, LT. "Flavonoids and cognitive function: a review of human randomized controlled trial studies and recommendations for future studies." *Genes and Nutrition*, (2009): 227-242.

26. Morris MC, Evans DA, Bienias JL, Tangney CC, Bennett DA, Aggarwal N, Schneider J, Wilson RS. "Dietary fats and the risk of incident Alzheimer disease." *Archives of Neurology*, (2003): 194-200.

27. Morris MC, Evans DA, Bienias JL, Tangney CC, Wilson RS. "Dietary fat intake and 6-year cognitive change in an older biracial community population." *Neurology*, (2004): 1573-1579.

Chapter 5

28. Krikorian R, Shidler MD, Nash TA, Kalt W, Vingyist-Tymchuk MR, Shukitt-Hale B, Joseph JA. "Blueberry supplementation improves memory in older adults." *Journal of Agricultural and Food Chemistry*, (2010): 3996-4000.

29. Cinta Valls-Pedret, Aleix Sala-Vila, Merce Serra-Mir. "Mediterranean diet and age-related cognitive decline – a randomized clinical trial." *Journal of the American Medical Association Internal Medicine*, (2015): 1094-1103.

30. Poulose SM, Miller MG, Shukitt-Hale B. "Role of walnuts in maintaining brain health with age." *The Journal of Nutrition*, (2014): 561S-566S.

31. Valls-Pedret C, Lamuela-Raventos RM, Medina-Remon A, et. al. "Polyphenol-rich foods in the Mediterranean diet are associated with better cognitive function in elderly subjects at high cardiovascular risk." *Journal of Alzheimer's Disease*, (2012): 773-782.

32. Willcox DC, Scapagnini G, Willcox BJ. "Healthy aging diets other than the Mediterranean: A focus on the Okinawan diet." *Mechanisms of Ageing and Development*, (2014): 148-162.

33. Shakersain B, Saritoni G, Larsson SC, Faxen-Irving G, Fastborn J, Fratiglioni L, Xu W. "Prudent diet may attenuate the adverse effects of Western diet on cognitive decline." *Alzheimer's and Dementia*, (2016): 100-109.

34. Fredrik Jerneren, Amany K, et. al. "Brain atrophy in cognitively impaired elderly: the importance of long-chain omega-3 fatty acids and B vitamin status in a randomized controlled trial." *The American Journal of Clinical Nutrition*, (2015): 215-221.

35. Fitzgerald S. "Seafood found neuroprotective for Alzheimer's in those with the risk gene." *Neurology Today*, (2016): 1,4-7.

36. O'Connor LE, Paddon-Jones D, Wright AJ, Campbell WW. "Mediterranean-style eating pattern with lean, unprocessed red meat has cardiometabolic benefits for adults who are overweight or obese in a randomized, crossover, controlled feeding trial." *The American Journal of Clinical Nutrition*, (2018): 33-40.

37. Roussell MA, Hill AM, Gaugler TL, West SG, et. al. "Beef in an optimal lean diet study: effects on lipids, lipoproteins, and apolipoproteins." *The American Journal of Clinical Nutrition*, (2012): 9-16.

38. Fernando WMADB, Martins IJ, Goozee KG, Brennan CS. "The role of dietary coconut for the prevention and treatment of Alzheimer's disease: potential mechanisms of action." *British Journal of Nutrition*, (2015): 1-14.

39. Yang Q, Zhang Z, Gregg EW, Flanders WD, Merritt R, Hu FB. "Added sugar intake and cardiovascular diseases mortality among US adults." *Journal of the American Medical Association of Internal Medicine*, (2014): 516-524.

40. Healthypeople.gov. 202 Objectives; Nutrition and Weight Status.

41. Snachez-Muniz FJ. "Oils and fats: change due to culinary and industrial processes." *International Journal for Vitamin and Nutrition Research*, (2006): 230-237.

Chapter 7

42. Bennett DA, Schneider JA, Arvanitakis Z, Wilson RS. "Overviewer and findings from the religious orders study." *Current Alzheimer's Research*, (2012): 628-645.

43. Bennett DA, Schneider JA, Buchman AS, Barnes LL, Boyle PA, Wilson RS. "Overview and findings from the rush memory and aging project." *Current Alzheimer's Research*, (2012): 646-63.

44. Hughes TF. "Promotion of cognitive health through cognitive activity in the aging population." *The Journal of Aging and Health*, (2010): 111-121.

45. Vidoni ED, Johnson DK, Morris JK, Van Sciver A, Greer CS, Billinger SA, Donnelly JE, Burns JM. "Dose-response of aerobic exercise on cognition: a community-based, pilot randomized controlled trial." *Plos One*, (2015).

46. Brinke LF, Bolandzadeh N, Nagamatsu LS, Hsu CL, Davis JC, Miran-Khan K, Liu-Ambrose T. "Aerobic exercise increases hippocampal volume in older women with probable mild cognitive impairment: a 6-month randomized controlled trial." *British Journal of Sports Medicine*, (2013).

47. Rehfeld K, Muller P, Aye N, Schmicker M, Dordevic M, Kaufmann J, Hokelmann A, Muller NG. "Dancing or fitness sport? The effects of two training programs on hippocampal plasticity and balance abilities in seniors." *Frontiers in Human Neuroscience*, (2017).

48. Cook Maher A, Kielb S, Loyer E, Connelley M, Rademaker A, Marsel Mesulam M, Weintraub S, McAdams D, Logan R, Rogalski E. "Psychological well-being in elderly adults with extraordinary episodic memory." *PLOS ONE*, (2017).

49. Patrick CJ. "Understanding the role of conscientiousness of healthy aging: Where does the brain come in?" *Developmental Psychology*, (2014):1465-1469.

50. Kaplin A, Anzaldi L. "New movement in neuroscience: A purpose-driven life." *Cerebrum*, (2015).

51. Levy BR, Slade MD, Pietrzak RH, Ferrucci L. "Positive age beliefs protect against dementia even among elders with high-risk gene." *PLOS One*, (2018).

INDEX

A

Alzheimer's disease 1-5, 7-15, 17, 20-21, 24-25, 28, 31, 33, 35, 37-38, 42, 45, 48, 53-54, 56, 59, 67-69, 72-74

Anthocyanins 24, 42

Antioxidants 16-17, 25, 32-34, 41, 43, 45, 49, 57, 76, 79-80, 83-84, 95-96, 99-100, 103, 107

B

B-vitamins 11, 25, 30-32, 50-51, 81, 83-84, 86

Beans 23, 40, 46-47, 61-65, 96, 103

Berries 22-25, 38, 41-42, 44, 62-63, 65-66, 75, 79, 80, 91, 95, 100, 107

Beta-amyloid 13, 15

Blood-brain barrier 18-19, 30

Brain 1-2, 4-5, 8, 10-26, 28, 30-43, 45-51, 53-54, 56-60, 62, 64, 67, 68-76, 79-81, 83-84, 86, 88, 91-92, 95-96, 99-100, 103-104, 107,

Brain draining foods 37, 53, 57

Brain healthy foods 22-23, 45, 53

Brain healthy lifestyle, guidelines 67

Brain sustaining foods 37-38

C

Carotenoids 33-34, 39-41, 58

Cholesterol 22, 47, 49, 52, 73, 75

Cognitive decline 11, 20-22, 30,-33, 35, 38-39, 41, 45, 47, 69-70, 73

D

DASH diet 21-22, 52

Dementia 3-5, 8-12, 20-22, 24-25, 38, 43, 49, 56, 67-68, 70, 72-73

Dementia with Lewy bodies 10

Dietary fat 35

Dietary Guidelines for Americans 44

E
Extra virgin olive oil 38, 49-50, 54, 65, 79, 92

F
Fast foods 57
Fiber 43, 46-47, 56, 75-76, 79-81, 83, 85-86, 88-89, 91-92, 95-96, 99-100, 103-104, 107
Fish 22-23, 25, 31, 36, 48, 51, 57-58, 61, 63-65, 73, 84
Flavonoids 33-35, 42
Folate 25, 30-32, 38, 75, 88, 92, 99
Fried foods 57-58
Fruits 24, 34-35, 41, 73, 100

H
Homocysteine 25, 31-32

I
Inflammation 13, 19, 24, 34-35, 42, 49, 53, 57, 69

L
Legumes 22, 46, 47, 73

M
Meal planning 59-62
Mediterranean diet 21-22, 38, 45
Meninges 16-18
Micronutrients 29, 58
Mild cognitive impairment 10-11
MIND diet 21-22, 24-25, 49-51, 54, 58, 73
Mixed dementia 10
Monounsaturated fat 35, 49, 52, 84, 99, 104, 107

N
Normal pressure hydrocephalus 3, 10
Nutrient density 30

O
Oils 25, 29, 32, 36, 48-50, 54, 64-65, 69
Omega-3 fatty acids 25, 36, 45, 48-49, 65, 80-81, 84, 86, 88, 92, 99-100, 104
Oxidative stress 16-17, 24-25, 33-34, 36, 42

P
Parkinson's disease 10
Pastries 24, 56-57

Polyunsaturated fats 35, 45, 48-49
Portion sizes 53, 62
Poultry 22-23, 31, 48, 50-51, 63-65, 81

R
Red meat 22, 24, 35, 48, 51-53, 63, 65

S
Saturated fats 22, 35, 45, 48-49
Sugary beverages 56-57
Sweets 22, 24, 56-57

T
Trans fat 53

U
Unhealthy foods 24
Unhealthy fats 53

V
Vascular dementia 10, 24-25
Vegetables 22-25, 34-36, 38-41, 49, 55, 63-66, 73, 89, 99

W
Whole grains 22-23, 43-44, 63, 65, 73
Whole fat cheeses 54-55

Made in the USA
Middletown, DE
01 April 2025

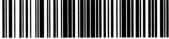

73619637R00076